Psychology and Social Action

Centennial Psychology Series
Charles D. Spielberger, *General Editor*

Psychology and Social Action

Selected Papers

Seymour B. Sarason

PRAEGER

PRAEGER SPECIAL STUDIES • PRAEGER SCIENTIFIC

Library of Congress Cataloging in Publication Data

Sarason, Seymour Bernard, 1919–
    Psychology and social action.

    (Centennial psychology series)
    Bibliography: p.
    Includes indexes.
    1. Community mental health services—Addresses,
essays, lectures. 2. Mental health—Addresses, essays,
lectures. 3. Psychology—Addresses, essays, lectures.
I. Title. II. Series.
RA790.5.S27   302   81-19944
ISBN 0-03-059332-8   AACR2

Published in 1982 by Praeger Publishers
CBS Educational and Professional Publishing
A Division of CBS, Inc.
521 Fifth Avenue, New York, New York 10017 U.S.A.

Printed in the United States of America

Contents

Editor's Introduction

The founding of Wilhelm Wundt's laboratory at Leipzig in 1879 is widely acclaimed as the landmark event that provided the initial impetus for the development of psychology as an experimental science. To commemorate scientific psychology's one-hundredth anniversary, Praeger Publishers commissioned the Centennial Psychology Series. The general goals of the Series are to present, in both historical and contemporary perspective, the most important papers of distinguished contributors to psychological theory and research.

As psychology begins its second century, the Series proposes to examine the foundation on which scientific psychology is built. Each volume provides a unique opportunity for the reader to witness the emerging theoretical insights of eminent psychologists whose seminal work has served to define and shape their respective fields, and to share with them the excitement associated with the discovery of new scientific knowledge.

The selection of the Series authors was an extremely difficult task. Indexes of scientific citations and rosters of the recipients of prestigious awards for research contributions were examined. Nominations were invited from leading authorities in various fields of psychology. The opinions of experienced teachers of psychology and recent graduates of doctoral programs were solicited. There was, in addition, a self-selection factor: a few of the distinguished senior psychologists invited to participate in the Series were not able to do so, most often because of demanding commitments or ill health.

Each Series author was invited to develop a volume comprising five major parts: (1) an original introductory chapter; (2) previously published articles and original papers selected by the author; (3) a concluding chapter; (4) a brief autobiography; and (5) a complete bibliography of the author's publications. The main content of each volume consists of articles and papers especially selected for this Series by the author. These papers trace the historical development of the author's work over a period of forty to fifty years. Each volume also provides a cogent presentation of the author's current research and theoretical viewpoints.

In their introductory chapters, Series authors were asked to describe the intellectual climate that prevailed at the beginning of their scientific careers and to examine the evolution of the ideas that led them from one study to another. They were also invited to com-

ment on significant factors—both scientific and personal—that stimulated and motivated them to embark on their research programs and
to consider special opportunities or constraints that influenced their
work, including experimental failures and blind alleys only rarely
reported in the literature. In order to preserve the historical record,
most of the articles reprinted in the Series volumes have been repro-
duced exactly as they appeared when they were first published. In
some cases, however, the authors have abridged their original papers
(but not altered the content), so that redundant materials could be
eliminated and more papers could be included.

In the concluding chapters, the Series authors were asked to
comment on their selected papers, to describe representative studies
on which they are currently working, and to evaluate the status of
their research. They were also asked to discuss major methodological
issues encountered in their respective fields of interest and to identify contemporary trends that are considered most promising for
future scientific investigation.

The biographical sketch that is included in each Series volume
supplements the autobiographical information contained in the original and concluding chapters. Perhaps the most difficult task faced
by the Series authors was selecting from the comprehensive bibliography a limited number of papers that they considered most representative of their life work.

Sarason's Contributions

Although general guidelines were suggested for each series volume,
each author was encouraged to adapt the Series format to meet his or
her own individual needs. The papers reprinted in this book reflect
Professor Sarason's major contributions to clinical and community
psychology, and readily attest to his significant role in founding and
helping to establish the latter field.

In his introductory chapter, Professor Sarason describes some of
the strongly held personal beliefs and implicit assumptions that
guided and shaped his productive career. His early theoretical convictions regarding enviornmental determinism, his abiding dissatisfaction with the status quo, and his deep personal commitment to
contributing to beneficial social change help us understand the evolution of his scientific research.

A major theme that underlies Sarason's work concerns the influence of social settings on psychological theory, research, and professional practice. This theme is vividly reflected in Sarason's description

of the pervasive impact on his later work of his first job at a new and innovative institution for the mentally retarded and in his transition in 1945 to the stimulating and challenging atmosphere of Yale's institute of Human Relations. Noting that many of the ideas expressed in his recent work were present in his early research on testing and mental retardation, Sarason observes that these insights could not be developed until they were shaped by the social changes of the 1960s and 1970s and until the climate within the field of psychology was more receptive.

Professor Sarason's early work on psychological testing and mental deficiency is represented in the first three papers in this Series volume. Psychologists familiar with his significant contributions to community psychology will find several papers that describe his creative insights into developing new settings, the powerful influence of community networks, and prescriptions for problem solving and social action. The absence of any papers on anxiety may be surprising to psychologists whose research in this area greatly benefited from the sophisticated theory, research, and measurement techniques generated during the 1950s by Sarason and his colleagues at Yale. Although Professor Sarason may place less value on this aspect of his productive career, his research continues to have tremendous impact and must be carefully studied by anyone interested in understanding the nature and measurement of anxiety and its effects on human behavior.

The personal beliefs and theoretical and philosophical assumptions that have guided Sarason's work are most clearly revealed in this volume in his papers criticizing psychology's continuing emphasis on the individual organism. Observing that American psychology has reflected the cultural impact of a particular society at a special time in its history, Professor Sarason argues forcefully that psychology needs to focus on real-world social problems and to intensify its commitment to facilitating constructive change through social action.

The Centennial Psychology Series is especially designed for courses on the history of psychology. Individual volumes are also well suited for use as supplementary texts in those areas to which the authors have been major contributors. Students of psychology and related disciplines, as well as authorities in specialized fields, will find that each Series volume provides penetrating insight into the work of a significant contributor to the behavioral sciences. The Series also affords a unique perspective on psychological research as a living process.

The interest and enthusiasm of all with whom we have consulted concerning the establishment of the Series have been most gratifying, but I am especially grateful to Professors Anne Anastasi, Hans J. Eysenck, and Irving L. Janis for their many helpful comments and suggestions and for their early agreement to contribute to the Series. For his invaluable advice and consultation in the conception and planning of the Series, and for his dedicated and effective work in making it a reality, I am deeply indebted to Dr. George Zimmar, psychology editor for Praeger Publishers. The Series was initiated while I was a Fellow-In-Residence at the Netherlands Institute for Advanced Study, and I would like to express my appreciation to the director and staff of the institute and to my NIAS colleagues for their stimulation, encouragement, and strong support of this endeavor.

Charles D. Spielberger

Psychology and Social Action

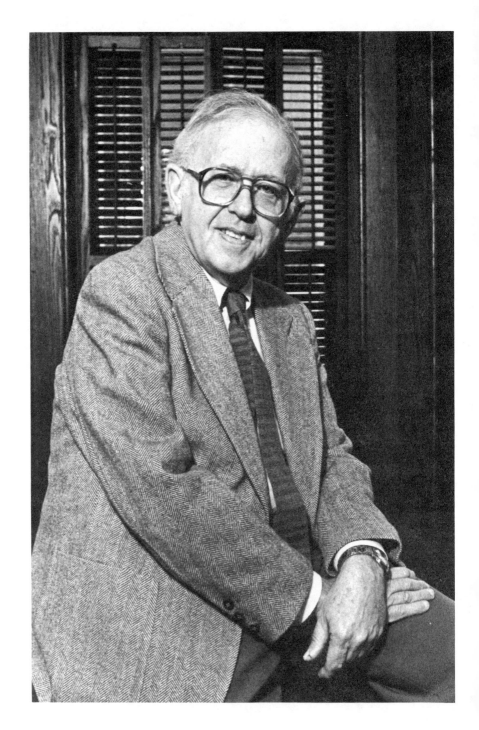

1

Introduction

Memory is a double-edged sword. If I had any doubts about that, they evaporated when I started to read what I had written over a period of forty years. I remembered the titles of the journal articles and, in a general way, their thrust, but I was amazed to find sentences, paragraphs, and sections containing ideas I thought I had come upon and developed only relatively recently. I do not think this is unusual. In the normal course of living, memory is rarely tested by confrontation with an objective record of the context from which the memory emerged. We are unaware, fortunately and unfortunately, how much myth is part of the memory. There is another explanation—not contradictory but complicating. An earlier version of an idea may sound remarkably similar to a later one, but the context in which the earlier one was embedded did not permit pursuit of the idea's implications. How can I explain how contexts and ideas changed? I do not pretend to be able to give a satisfactory answer to that question, but I believe I can identify some of the answer's ingredients.

The first ingredient is perhaps the clearest: when I started out, I already had the conviction that our society was organized in ways that made it extraordinarily difficult for people to develop their capacities—impossible for most people. As a Marxist (Trotskyite version), a Jew, a physically handicapped person—and someone who was massively affected by the Great Depression—I was predisposed to be partisan to the underdog and to be an opponent of the status quo. This was an extreme environmentalist stance, but whatever its oversimplifications it sensitized me to the importance of micro and macro social contexts. It never really made sense to me to focus on the individual, to explain his or her behavior in individual terms. What was fateful for me in this stance was its commitment to action for

1

the purposes of change. I was not content to understand people and
the social world—I wanted to change them—and I did not see change
in narrow, clinically interpersonal terms. As a clinical psychologist, I
enjoyed working with individuals, but I always saw the individual in
some adversary relationship to the social surround.

In the early days, I did not articulate this first ingredient well. It
was more in the nature of a *weltanschauung*—largely a melange of un-
articulated beliefs and assumptions that possessed me more than I
possessed them. The second ingredient provided the context for
somewhat clearer articulation. My first professional job after finishing
graduate school in 1942 was as psychologist in a new, innovative
state institution for the mentally retarded. I knew that the mentally
retarded were rejected by society, that a significant number of them
were of the Kallikak variety whose genes were supposed to be of inferior quality, and that society tended to view the retarded as a burden and interference from whom society would receive no benefit
whatsoever. The Southbury Training School provided me with the
context in which to demonstrate the thrust of my weltanschauung. I
became a partisan for mentally retarded people. I saw them in an institutional context whose organization and characteristics tended to
be inimical to the recognition of their capacities and to my efforts to
alter the context. Most of the ideas that I developed more fully later
in my career germinated during my years at Southbury, but that context was too restricted for me to see the more general significance of
those ideas. As the residents of this institution in the middle of the
beautiful Connecticut nowhere were socially and intellectually restricted, so was my thinking similarly bounded by that setting. Whatever I experienced and learned had meaning in and for that context,
a limitation of which I was then unaware. This limitation was enor-
mously helpful to me, however, precisely because working *and* living
in such an isolated setting enabled me—indeed forced me—to recognize
how the behavior of individuals (residents and staff) varied as a function of the structure of the various settings contained in the institution. I came to see how inadequate, distracting, and even harmful
psychological test scores and diagnostic labels could be for recognizing and comprehending behavioral-performance variations in different institutional contexts. After all, if you know and have commerce with almost every human being in the institution, if you see
almost all of them in a variety of contexts, it is hard not to recognize
the limitations of labels.

A third ingredient that helps account for how contexts and ideas
changed was my leaving Southbury and going to Yale. Elsewhere I
have described the personal, social, and intellectual significance of
that transition:

I was a psychologist the day I left Southbury, and I was the "same" psychologist when I came to Yale, but the identity of public labels hid the fact that I was seeking rebirth. And here I must relate something which casts a different light over all that I have said so far. It is not only relevant to how one thinks about jobs and careers but also to the issue of candor and the one life–one career imperative.

When Esther and I left the chairman's home in a New Haven suburb, having come to final agreement about the offer and my acceptance, evening had come together with a spring mist which made the blooming dogwoods (in which the area abounds) look unusually heavy. We had about three blocks to walk to the bus. We never took the bus. When we left the chairman's house we said not a word to each other for about a minute, we just walked hand-in-hand. Then, as if by some prearranged signal, we turned to each other and shouted: "We are free!" That utterance was the first time I had allowed myself to say something out loud that reflected vague fears about spending our social lives in an institutional setting, and being intellectually confined by having to focus on a particular patient population. There was a part of me that knew that by coming to Southbury the confines of my career had already been determined: my positions might change, my status and income increase, I would write and do research, and I would try to branch out, but all of this would be as a clinical psychologist in a state institutional setting. When I day-dreamed about all the great and wonderful things I would do in my lifetime, the physical setting in which these would be done was a Southbury or one of its different kin. For the first two years at Southbury I enjoyed these daydreams. I was lucky, I had it made! I had *a* career line, thank God. I knew what my life would be like, and I liked the prospect. If anyone had told me that I was uncriticaly buying the one life–one career imperative, I would have signed his commitment papers. It was after a couple of years, and it was only in part a function of my marriage, that I would have fleeting and disquieting thoughts about what the long-term future looked like. But I never really allowed myself to pursue these thoughts. Where would it get me? Besides, wasn't I learning and doing a lot, and wasn't there a lot more to do? What more did I want? Sure, institutional life and work leave something to be desired, but you have to put these negatives in perspective. I never could bring myself to discuss this openly with anyone, particularly with Esther, who never hesitated to tell me how she regarded institutional living. I resented her putting into words what I feared to let myself think about. Why get upset about what you cannot alter? I saw the future and accommodated to it. So when we walked into freedom upon leaving the chairman's home, masculine me could for the first time acknowledge what I had previously allowed (= required) myself to believe was weakness and irrationality. I had been in prison and thought it was freedom. Relative to any other institution I knew or heard about, I did have freedom at Southbury; relative to Yale it was a concentration camp. (Sarason, 1977, 1)

I carried a lot of Southbury with me to Yale but now I was seeing what I had experienced and learned in a very different context. It was not only that I was now part of a challenging and stimulating atmosphere that inevitably broadened my knowledge of psychology, forcing me to examine and relate my ideas to other points of view and bodies of knowledge, but I also had to teach—to profess. Few activities rival teaching in the demands it makes on examination and reexamination of how you think. To me, it is like being a witness in a courtroom. You not only have to be clear about what you are saying, but you have to be prepared to justify your testimony and to meet challenges to it. There was no shortage of challenges, indirect and direct. The indirect challenge came from the simple fact that I was surrounded by a collection of high-powered social scientists whose thinking and writing I needed to comprehend if I was to be a functioning member of the setting. When I came to Yale in 1945, the Institute of Human Relations housed the departments of psychology and psychiatry, part of the department of anthropology (for example, Linton and Murdock), the child development centers headed by Arnold Gesell, and the labor-management center (for example, Bakke and Argyris). I was exposed to and challenged by more ideas and people than I could absorb, except over a period of years. The direct challenge came from graduate students, some of whom were as old or older than I and no less capable. For ten years after World War II, the quality of graduate students, many of whom had spent years in the armed forces, was amazing. They were not shrinking violets, and to a young assistant professor they were intimidating. In my teaching I drew, of course, on my Southbury experience, but in ways known and unknown to me the significances of that experience were changing. There is another aspect to this ingredient that can be too easily overlooked: Yale is not a campus college; it is in the "Broadway and Forty-second Street" area of New Haven. To someone like me, just coming from rural Connecticut, it was back in the real world—and what was the relevance for that world of what I had learned at Southbury? I do not think I ever asked myself that question, but with the advantage of hindsight it is as if the development of my thinking was powered by that question. I have no doubt that, if I had gone to a nonurban university instead of going to Yale, the ideas that germinated at Southbury would have had a different development, and some would have had no further development at all. The transition from Southbury to urban Yale had the effect (again unknown to me) of underlining something I had learned at Southbury—that it is hard to overestimate the influences of the social-geographical surround. This explains why, early on, I came to regard Roger Barker's work with such respect. Unfortunately, he has had little influence on the development of modern psychology. To someone unacquainted with his work, I suggest starting with a chapter ("The Influence of Frontier Environments on Behavior") that he contributed to *The American West: New Perspectives, New Dimensions* (Steffen, 1979). I knew Barker's work long before I was able to use it, and I was only able to use it when I was able to replay past experience and see it afresh.

The fourth ingredient was the most impersonal and uncontrollable at the same time that it was the most fateful. World War II changed the world more quickly and pervasively than any previous event or war. You cannot understand the major stories in today's newspaper without coming to grips with the origins and consequences of World War II. We like to say that we live in an era of fast and bewildering change, and until a few years ago change was synonymous with progress, which is why some people gave themselves badges of honor for accommodating to change. For reasons not at all clear to me, I never felt comfortable with the conceptions of either change or progress. I have always been fascinated with social and intellectual history, and there was a good deal in what I read (and observed) to suggest that our western world was born a long time ago and that, despite the obvious and dramatic ways in which science and technology have been used to change that world, the changes were in the service of a world view that had not changed very much. World War II did usher in an era of enormous change, which was hard not to believe, given the force and frequency of that message in the mass media. The world of today, to somebody who grew up in the pre–World War II era, is a remarkably changed place. If the world has changed that much, however, why are the problems (nationalism, war, racism, religious conflict, competing political ideologies, poverty, and so on) that beset the world so remarkably similar, in substance if not in degree, to what they were fifty or a hundred years ago? It is not necessary for the reader to agree with me, because the point I want to make is that I am a person who does not easily give up on ideas that grip me (a mixed blessing, I know), especially if they involve distinctions between appearance and reality, between phenotype and genotype. I have come to this view of myself relatively late in life.

Thus, there was a part of me that should not have been surprised when I saw in my early papers ideas that did not get developed until many years had gone by. Now I know—now I can see—that almost everything I have ever written had its conceptual origins in the Southbury experience. There was Southbury, and all else had been commentary. That commentary was sustained, however, by the peculiar relationship between the major issues in the field of mental retardation and the societal dynamics unleashed by World War II. Race, poverty, civil rights, segregation (educational and otherwise), urban decay, community resources and responsibility, the population explosion, the dawning of the "age of mental health"—as these issues emerged into the arena of public discussion and policy, it was inevitable that the field of mental retardation would begin to receive attention. I was convinced of that—a conviction that became an obsession during my first three years at Yale, when my eyes were opened to other social sciences. Psychology is a social science, but then (and now) graduate education in psychology was a parochial affair. Yale's Institute of Human Relations enabled me to expand my knowledge of other social sciences, particularly anthropology. The influence of that setting is obvious in my first book, *Psychological Problems in Mental Deficiency* (1949,1). If I was convinced that mental retardation was a window through which to see the workings of society, I had few supporters. Who was interested in mental retardation? Schizophrenia, neurosis, and psychoanalysis were the attractive issues of the day. In fact, my publisher agreed to publish the book only if I would accept reduced royalties on the first 2,500 copies. Even then they expected to lose money, but in those days—when publishers were beginning to benefit financially from the consequences of the GI Bill, of which millions of veterans were taking advantage—the publisher was willing to risk some loss on a book in an esoteric area. The subsequent history of that book surprised them, but not me. In writing that book I thought I had milked dry my Southbury experience, but, as it turned out, the Southbury experience informed everything I did subsequently. The work in the dozen or more years I spent with the Test Anxiety Project can be directly traced to things I wrote in that first book on mental retardation. My involvement in starting the Yale Psycho-Educational Clinic and in helping to develop the field of community psychology was a direct consequence of the Southbury experience (Sarason, 1966, 4; 1979, 1). My book *The Creation of Settings and the Future Societies* (1972, 1) explicitly derives from my preoccupation with how a new setting, such as the Southbury Training School, fails in its purposes. The important point here is less the Southbury experience than the fact that the social world changed in ways that made me continue to reflect on and utilize that experience. To the extent that I could continue to make sense of the Southbury experience, I was making sense of the larger society. That was the unverbalized assumption that seemed to guide me.

The final ingredient has to do with the benefits and tortures of writing. Writing is torture for me because, as soon as I take pencil to paper, I realize that I have not been thinking in any concentrated, critical way, except for perhaps two or three minutes at a time. The ideas are there—in a strange mixture of visual imagery, words, and phrases, and emotional excitement—but that mixture does not get the writing started. I pick up the pencil and immediately realize that ideas are horribly complex and that language is like the sculptor's stone—it is massively there, challenging me, defying me to select the right beginning point, to follow through, chipping here, chipping there, always aware that the creator and the material must undergo reciprocal changes. Nothing makes me more humble about the clarity of my ideas than trying to represent them in written language. The task becomes even more problematic if you believe, as I do, that everything is or can be related to everything else. What do I leave out, what should be the central focus, how could I not have seen this or that connection? The benefits are inherent in the tortures, however. Writing is learning, unlearning, reliving—a discovery process about myself and the problem. Figure and ground are always changing, and frequently what gets relegated to ground—still there, related to the figure, but not what will force itself on the reader—are ideas that get no independent development. The writer may consider them important, but it is unlikely that the reader will.

This book is supposed to trace the development of my thinking. As I read what I have just written, I realize that I am uncomfortable with the concept of development, if that means a continuous, somewhat self-conscious, self-directed process in the course of which ideas are broadened and transformed, albeit containing threads of continuity. Such a concept of development does not fit my phenomenology. On the contrary, I see myself as someone who reacted to events and problems external to me; only after reacting for a time could I find something in my past to relate to what I was experiencing. The continuity only became apparent *after* I had immersed myself in events and problems and *after* I had taken pencil to paper to make sense of what I experienced. I lust for experience, but not because I am compelled by anything resembling clear ideas whose validity I want to establish. Rationality and systematic preparatory thinking are not distinguishing features of my development. The major distinguishing feature is a need to make sense of my experiences, to order them, but the intervals between the emergence of that need contain a great deal of experiencing and remarkably little systematic thinking.

With one possible exception, the ideas contained in this book have been expressed by others, but neither they nor I have influenced mainstream psychology. I was pleased to have been asked to contribute to this series, but my pleasure had nothing to do with an over-

estimation of my influence on the field and a good deal to do with
the opportunity to have another forum to state where I have stood
and where I stand. I have influenced individuals but not the fields of
which I have been a part. That was to be expected, because so much
of what I have written addresses and requires social change. American
psychology has never faced up to the fact that it is the creation of a
particular society, bearing in many ways the world view of that society. Psychology has maintained the fiction that the substance of
its theories and the pictures of man that they project are independent
of the relationship of the theorists to the social order. Psychologists
have never been a random sampling of the population, but the implications of that obvious fact have yet to be confronted. American
psychology has been quintessentially a psychology of the individual
organism, with society vaguely, even inchoately, in the background.
So long as psychology was a small, university-based field in the pre-
World War II era, the limitations of the focus on the individual organisms were not apparent. When psychology entered the real world
after World War II, however, full of promise for contributing to a re-
fashioning of the social order (national and international) and eager
to establish its centrality to the problems of social change, the stage
was set for the current malaise among psychologists. The reader who
is too young to have experienced the optimism about psychology in
the decade or so after World War II will have difficulty in grasping
the stark contrast in outlook between then and now. To begin to
understand that contrast is, I believe, the most important problem
that psychology as science and profession has to face. Not until
psychology recognizes the limitations of its focus on the individual
organism will it recognize how much a reflection it has been of a
particular society at a particular time in its history. In articulating
that view in my most recent book *Psychology Misdirected: The Psychologist in the Social Order* (1981, 1), I have returned to where I
started—the social-historical process. My socialization into psychology
obscured and diverted me from the importance of that process. That
is no cause for regret, because I was then far less prepared to think
about that process than I am now; and I am still very ill prepared.

The reader will note that most of the articles in this book come
from the last fifteen years. I have not included a single paper from
the many that came out of the Test Anxiety Project over a dozen
years ago, beginning in the late 1940s. That project was interpersonally rewarding and, by any set of conventional criteria, unusually
productive and successful. The fact is, however, that the project
contributed amazingly little to my intellectual development. It
helped make me known in psychology, it demonstrated I could do

empirical research, and it certainly helped me get tenure and promotions at Yale. Since this collection is supposed to contain papers that I regard as indicative of growth (if not linear development), however, I could not include a single study from the Test Anxiety Project. I hasten to add that, if I could start all over again, I would not leave that project out, because it was one of two times in my adult life (the Yale Psycho-Educational Clinic period was the other) when I was surrounded by so many decent, sensitive, bright people. I needed and experienced the psychological sense of community long before I ever conceptualized and wrote about it in *The Psychological Sense of Community: Prospects for a Community Psychology* (1974). It was not by chance that that book was written after I left the directorship of the clinic—after I could come to terms with the personal significance of the clinic years and after I knew what I was no longer experiencing.

REFERENCE

Steffen, J. O. (Ed.) *The American West: New perspectives, new dimensions.* Norman: University of Oklahoma Press, 1979.

Commentary to
Chapter 2

*I knew the young lady discussed in this paper in two very different
contexts: the formal, standardized testing situation and a hospital
laboratory. In the former she appears far less adequate than the latter,
although I try (strain) to indicate which aspects of her test performance should be viewed as cautions against underestimating her
capacities. As a young clinical psychologist whose major institutional
function was diagnostic testing, I was eager to demonstrate the util-
ity of new and old approaches to testing. Thus, rather than trying to
explain what there was about the social context of the hospital
laboratory that permitted the productive learning I describe, I concentrate on the interpretation of her test behavior and performance.
I was focusing on her as an individual, not on the contexts of which
she was a part. What is the nature of problem-solving behavior in
naturally occurring (or noncontrived) contexts, and what relationship does the quality and level of that behavior have to problem
solving in formal, standardized testing situations? That was the important, albeit poorly formulated question that forced itself upon me
from the day I started to work at the Southbury Training School. On
that day I found myself part of a "posse" looking for a profoundly
retarded individual who had run away from the institution. How could
an individual who had an IQ in the forties plan and execute a successful runaway? What amazed me when I reread this paper was the following sentence: "A more recent manifestation of the limitations of
the intelligence test results is the number of so-called defectives who
have not only successfully adjusted to the Armed Services program
but who have also become noncommissioned officers and in some
instances been cited for bravery." Now I know why, years later, in
writing my part of the Sarason and Gladwin monograph* Psychological and Cultural Problems in Mental Subnormality* (1958, 6), I was so
happy to come across Ginzberg and Bray's 1953 book* The Unedu-
cated, containing detailed descriptions of the problem-solving
behavior of low test-scoring individuals in situations of battle stress.
In 1980 I wrote a review of Jensen's* Bias in Mental Testing.* In it I
say: "From my standpoint, the Achilles heel in Jensen's position, as
well in those of his critics, is the significance they attach to standardized tests and testing conditions. The question I wish to discuss is:
what is the relation between problem solving in test situations and*

*in non-contrived, naturally occurring situations?" I conclude the
review as follows:*

> The question I am raising goes far beyond mental testing. Indeed, it has
> been explicitly raised by a highly sophisticated group of experimental
> cognitive psychologists led by Michael Cole at Rockefeller University. I
> refer specifically to their monograph bearing the delightful title: *Ecologi-
> cal niche picking: ecological invalidity as an axiom of experimental cogni-
> tive psychology.* On the basis of their studies of test and non-test behavior
> these researchers are forced to the conclusion that at the present time
> " . . . laboratory models preclude the operation of principles essential to
> the organization of behavior in non-laboratory environments [and that]
> theories and data derived from the laboratory cannot be used as a basis
> for predictions about the behavior of individuals once they leave the
> laboratory."
>
>   Cole's studies and conclusions should be alarming both to Jensen and
> his critics because it points to a severe limitation, and possible semi-lethal
> defect, in the practice of validating performance in one standardized test-
> ing situation by another. I raised this issue a quarter of a century ago and
> Cole has raised it again in a more systematic, data-based way. Some day,
> perhaps, psychologists will start looking at performance in naturally
> occurring situations. That will be the day! (Sarason, 1980, 2)

*I did raise the issue clearly a quarter of a century ago, but I had
raised it unclearly thirty-seven years ago!*

*   I also must point out the parochial view of history this paper
reflects. Although it does reflect my abiding interest in history, it
is not the kind of social-intellectual history the problem requires.
Why was the Binet test so enthusiastically taken over and applied by
American psychology? Why was there such devotion to the concept
of objectivity? What did the institutional uses of tests say about how
our society was ordered and about the values underlying that order?
How do you explain fashions in psychology? The fact is that in this
paper I am talking about psychology as if it were independent of the
society from which it emerged, as if psychologists were not willing
agents of the world view of that society. I was too well socialized
into psychology to take distance from it.*

2

Projective Techniques in Mental Deficiency
The Relationship of Intelligence and Personality in the Study of the Mentally Deficient: Historical

Clinical psychology in the past has provided techniques for measuring behavior which have been taken over by the field of mental deficiency. The Binet is only one of such contributions. There are, however, definite disadvantages to this borrowing against which one must guard. One disadvantage lies in the fact that the field of psychology has been in a state of flux for many years so that what was once accepted may have been later rejected. A test may have remained the same, but its interpretive significance changed. From time to time new "schools of psychology" have gained ascendancy, their tenets percolating through the entire field, only to give way later to another school with newer insights. As the field matured, the differences between the schools became less distinct. Clinical psychology has not been uninfluenced by these developments. One may well ask, therefore, to what extent the field of mental deficiency has benefited from the increasing maturity of clinical psychology. An answer to this question requires a brief review of the clinical approach since 1916.

When the Binet tests came into use, personality and intelligence were implicitly considered divisible. That is, it was felt that one could objectively measure intellectual functioning apart from personality organization. One had merely to be instructed in administering and

S. B. Sarason, "Projective Techniques in Mental Deficiency," *Journal of Personality* (1944): 237–245. Copyright 1944 by the American Psychological Association. Reprinted by permission.

scoring the Binet in order to be judged competent to obtain a quotient or mental age which stood for an individual's intelligence. "I.Q." became a popular expression. The Binet was invested with a validity which few questioned. Since psychology had long been accused of being a subjective, nonscientific discipline, the relatively well-standardized 1916 Binet was welcomed as the fulfillment of the hopes of many. In some minds standardization and validity were synonymous. It was in this atmosphere that the Binet was accepted by workers in the field of mental deficiency and applied on a wholesale scale. Countless studies appeared in which the Binet was assumed to have given an accurate and complete picture not only of intellectual functioning but of capacity as well. The Binet became the basis for admission to institutions, and some workers had enough confidence in the test to set a certain intelligence quotient as a criterion below which a person could be considered feebleminded and above which he was presumably not.

The field of personality measurement in this early period was likewise dominated by the desire to be "objective" above all else. Attempts to construct paper-and-pencil tests in which statements which seemed to fit the patient were checked became standard practice. Rating scales and questionnaires were the vogue. It was fashionable at that time to group responses to standard questions so that an individual could be "typed." Workers in the field of mental deficiency also became imbued with this seemingly objective approach.

This early period of clinical psychology might be characterized as one in which human behavior was atomistically and mathematically approached. That which could not be observed or statistically measured was eschewed. The ultimate hope of many seemed to be the representation of behavior on a well-constructed graph. Man had finally achieved the dignity of a symbol in a formula.

The reaction against clinical atomism was not long in the coming and was a natural outcome of the extreme behaviorism demonstrated in the early period. The reaction was due largely to the impact of psychoanalysis, gestalt psychology, and the personalistic school. The uniqueness of any given individual's personality, the inextricable relationship between intelligence and personality, and the presence and motivating power of unconscious activity and striving were brought to the fore. It became clear that the intellectual functioning of an individual was subject to so many personality factors that any numerical representation of such functioning was bound to be a misrepresentation. It became apparent that a basic problem in clinical psychology was the development of means for determining the difference and relationship between capacity and functioning. Intelligence test results, acknowledged as valuable, came to be regarded as but one important manifestation of an individual's total functioning.

As a result of the psychoanalytic orientation a new technique for obtaining personality data came into greater use. This new technique was termed projective because the patient is allowed, unbeknown to himself, to bring forth his inner needs, desires, and conflicts. Information which ordinarily would not be revealed because of conscious suppression or unconscious repression could be elicited by the projective technique. New light was thrown on the subtle relationship between affect and intelligence. The most widely used of such techniques are the Rorschach ink-blot test and Murray's Thematic Apperception Test. Although many questions have been raised about the validity of the interpretation of these tests, there can be little doubt that they represent a distinct contribution to clinical psychology.

When one examines the psychological procedures employed at present with the mental defective, one still finds an overwhelming emphasis on the problem of intelligence measurement. The Binet, the 1916 or 1937 revision, is still used in the majority of cases as the sole basis for commitment to an institution. There has been very little clinical recognition of the fact that the defective child has as many problems of personality adjustment as the normal child. There has been little recognition of the fact that the intellectual level of the defective child may be depressed because of his maladjustments. Indeed, it is a real question as to how many of our so-called defectives have capacities which are normal in nature but which have been hidden by a variety of personality and social factors. It is doubtful that an approach which views intelligence only in terms of intelligence test quotients can ever answer the complicated problem of evaluating intellectual potentiality as distinguished from intellectual functioning.

AN ILLUSTRATIVE EXAMPLE

There have been many who have recognized the limitations of the standard tests of intelligence with the mental defective. For example, those who have observed for any length of time the mental defective in institutions have been struck time and again by the discrepancy in certain cases between the social functioning of the individual and his obtained general mental level or intelligence quotient. The most striking example the writer has seen is a seventeen-year-old girl at the Southbury Training School who was initially assigned to the hospital laboratory to do the simplest of routine tasks. The following are the results of tests given this girl:

Terman-Merrill (L)	M.A. 10–6	I.Q. 70
Arthur Point Scale	M.A. 10–11	I.Q. 73
Rorschach Achievement		
Reading	Grade 3.9	Age 9–3
Arithmetic	Grade 4.9	Age 10–4
Spelling	Grade 3.0	Age 8–3

After one year of training the girl was able to perform the following tasks:

1. Sterilization and chemical cleansing of glassware used in bacteriology and quantitative chemistry
2. Preparation of bacterial media, physiological and chemical solutions used in bacteriology, hematology, and qualitative chemistry
3. Cleansing of volumetric, graduated, and hematological pipettes and special chemical filters
4. Complete urinalysis except for microscopic including qualitative and quantitative sugars, albumin, acetone tests, and specific gravity
5. Streaking and plating of bacterial cultures with aseptic technique
6. Assistance in quantitative blood and tissue chemistry as in total proteins, lipids, sodiums, and potassiums
7. Staining of hematology and bacterial slides
8. Taking stool cultures and finger blood tests alone
9. Keeping daily record of work performed
10. All blood typing (all work is, of course, checked by head of the laboratory).

This girl's development has caused a good deal of surprise with those for whom she has worked. At the present time she is being instructed in the use of the microscope, and the State Health Laboratory has expressed a desire to employ her as a laboratory helper.

There are several qualitative and quantitative signs on the intelligence tests which suggest that this girl's capacity is higher than the obtained general mental level. Qualitatively one could safely say that the girl had much anxiety and insecurity during the examination. For example, when she was given the memory for designs item on the Binet, she very quickly and inaccurately scribbled some designs which had no relationship to the originals. Questioning revealed that she thought she was to reproduce the designs as quickly as possible. When given another piece of paper and told that speed was not a factor, she did noticeably better. This girl's desire to impress and achieve was so strong that even before directions for a task were completed she would nod her head knowingly, although it became evident that her anxiety about her ability to comprehend everything that was said prevented full comprehension. It is not surprising, therefore, to find this girl's performance on memory items variable, with a tendency to be poor. On problems involving sustained reasoning this girl performed above her obtained mental level—passing verbal absurdities at eight, nine, and eleven years, and the problem-of-fact and plan-of-search items at thirteen years. In reasoning problems this girl had such difficulty expressing her ideas that she stammered a good deal, became upset, and had to be encouraged often in order to calm her and to obtain a clear response. For example, it was approximately six minutes before she was able to express clearly her thoughts concerning the second verbal absurdity at eleven years. Another indication that this girl's capacity is probably higher than her obtained mental level is seen in the unusual quality of the words found in her spontaneous, conversational speech. On the Binet she was able to define abstract words on a fourteen-year level. On the Arthur performance scale, a non-verbal situation, this girl showed less anxiety than on the Binet. It should be noted that her lowest scores were on a test of conceptual thinking (Kohs block designs) and memory (Knox cube). On the Kohs designs she performed much below the obtained Binet or Arthur mental ages. The conclusions that may be drawn from this girl's performance on intelligence tests are that her functioning is variable in efficiency, that her capacity would seem to be higher than the obtained Binet mental age, and that personality factors hinder efficient display of her abilities. The obtained I.Q. or M.A. cannot be considered revealing of this girl's capacity since there are many who have obtained similar scores without a similar surprising development.

Without entering into a technical discussion, it can be said that this girl's creativeness, drive, and potentiality are more clearly in evidence in her Rorschach than in her intelligence-test performance. She organized the amorphous ink blots very well, regardless of whether she was using the whole blot or part of it. There was a distinct tendency, however, to use the whole blot in preference to parts of it, a characteristic which correlates with her everyday attempts to grasp intellectually as much as she can. She was not satisfied with the poor form of the blots but attempted to improve upon them, and her embellishments definitely enhanced the form accuracy of her responses. Several of her responses revealed a creative imagination since she was able to project human-like movement onto the cards. The estimate of this girl's intelligence from the Rorschach is much closer to her actual functioning than the picture gained from the Binet. The personality organization revealed by the Rorschach indicates that this girl has difficulty in overtly expressing herself emotionally and in smoothly responding to personal contact. The record contains constrictive qualities which increase her emotional problem. It is as if this girl approaches the environment in a fearful, cautious, stilted manner until her feelings of insecurity have been allayed by a friendly, accepting atmosphere. As is not unusual with the institutionalized child, the background of this girl was marked by neglect, economic privation, promiscuous and alcoholic parents, a broken home, and a lack of any source of discipline.

DISCUSSION

A more recent manifestation of the limitations of the intelligence test results is the number of so-called defectives who have not only successfully adjusted to the Armed Services' program but who also have become noncommissioned officers and in some instances been cited for bravery. While it is true that there are many defectives who have been inadequate in the Armed Services, the fact still remains that the intelligence quotient is unilluminating in regards to the reasons for success or failure of defectives of similar mental level.

An attempt to correct for the emphasis placed on intelligence testing is seen in Doll's Social Maturity Scale. This scale takes into account the social functioning of the individual, and in many cases the obtained picture is closer to our observations than any numerical result from an intelligence test. It should be noted, however, that in such a scale personality organization plays a minor role. While Doll's scale allows one to describe better the discrepancy between intellectual and social factors, it does not allow one to relate such a discrepancy to the personality organization of the individual.

A survey of the literature in mental deficiency would substantiate the layman's opinion that the mental defective is a dull, uninteresting, uncomplicated individual who, in layman terminology "doesn't have personality." It is surprising to note how few studies have appeared in which a single defective individual has been studied intensively so that his everyday intellectual and social functioning have been related to his hopes, fears, anxieties, and frustrations. The dearth of intensive, single-case studies is not paralleled in other fields where the psychologist and psychiatrist have applied themselves.

Apropos of the present discussion is the recent issue (September, 1944) of the *Journal of Counsulting Psychology* in which clinical psychologists from different types of hospitals discuss the duties and perspectives of psychologists in these agencies. It is noteworthy that in all but one of ten articles the Rorschach or Thematic Apperception tests are discussed as an important part of the psychologist's test battery. Equally interesting is the fact that there is no article on the duties of the clinical psychologist in state training schools and hospitals for the mentally defective—despite the fact that clinical psychology was greatly stimulated in its early phases by work with the feebleminded. It would seem that psychological work with the mental defective is regarded as dull and as routine as the defective himself.

Projective techniques have as yet been used to a very limited degree with mental defectives. What work has been done indicates that studies in the personality of the defective will be as rewarding and as interesting as work with any other group. However, some of the more extensive Rorschach studies with the feebleminded have not been too discriminating in the selection of subjects on the basis of common etiology. The term "feebleminded" or "mental defective" obscures the fact that there are many different etiologies for the condition. As with the term "insanity," one must be careful to differentiate one etiological group from another and not to mix them together in order to obtain the "typical" picture. With a discriminating use of controls projective techniques may well be found to be the means of filling the large gap that exists in our knowledge of the defective individual's feelings, needs, frustrations, and anxieties. If by the projective approach the total personality of the defective individual can be obtained, one may be better able to understand the basic problem of the relationship between potential and actual functioning.

It has been the custom to attribute much of the defective's behavior to the fact of his intellectual deficiency. Such a cause-and-effect approach seems to be an oversimplified formulation which neglects many factors. It would seem that clinical psychology in mental deficiency, possessed already of a "mature intelligence," is ready now for the acquisition of a "mature personality."

Projective techniques in mental deficiency should not receive the gullible acceptance that was true of the Binet. Recognition should be given the fact that projective techniques have not been thought by their proponents to be capable of the statistical refinement characteristic of intelligence tests. There is some question as to the feasibility and desirability of reducing the kind of data obtained from the Rorschach or Thematic Apperception tests to numerical scores. Although the administration and scoring of these tests are fairly well standardized, the interpretation of the tests, depending as it does on the experience and training of the clinician, requires cautious use and further study. For these reasons, the tests should be initially applied to carefully selected etiological groupings of such number that the individual case is not lost sight of in a maze of means, standard deviations, and critical ratios.

Results obtained on these tests from normal groups must not necessarily serve as validating criteria for data obtained from defectives. It should constantly be kept in mind that the defective child has usually had an unfortunate personal, social, and economic background, and encountered environmental pitfalls to which most normals have not been subjected. As a result, the defective child, especially the institutionalized one, more often than not, approached the test situation with fear, timidity, anxiety, or a feigned indifference; and the clinical psychologist must employ all his "psychology" if he is to get from the defective child maximum effort and representative functioning. For example, it is standard procedure on the Rorschach for the subject, after he has told the examiner the different things he has seen in each of the ten cards, to be questioned as to where on the card he saw what he did, and what it was about the blot that made him think of it. It became apparent in the writer's work with institutionalized defective children, however, that when the patient was asked to point out precisely the section of the blot he was using, he would sometimes become vague, uncertain, and unable to make up his mind. If the examiner should finally point to a section of the blot and ask if it were being used in the response, suggestibility might well be manifested. Such reactions might be interpreted as being either the result of intellectual deficiency and/or the result of the fact that one is dealing with the much-tested child who is conscious of the importance of the "brain test" and is fearful of giving the wrong answer. Some light is thrown on this problem by the fact that if before any questions are asked the child is told to trace what he sees, less indecisiveness is shown and one obtains a clearer picture of what was intended than if questions are asked which may be interpreted by the child as indicating that the response was incorrect.

Projective techniques are no panaceas for psychological problems in mental deficiency, and they are not intended as such. They are not substitutes for present methods but are additional tools which will throw much light upon the complicated relationship between functioning and capacity. The main contribution of the projective technique to the study of the defective individual is that it allows one to study the total personality and not merely isolated intellectual aspects of functioning.

Commentary to
Chapter 3

This article reflected my continuing interest in why predictions from test situations were so poor. Those were the days when diagnostic testing preoccupied clinical psychologists, but that was also a time when the successful prediction of behavior was regarded as a major criterion by which to judge psychology as a science. This article was the direct result of my having finished Psychological Problems in Mental Deficiency *(1949, 1), because, in thinking through and writing that book, I concluded that the "from what to what" prediction question was not being taken seriously. I regarded this article as a glimpse of the obvious, at the same time that I was suggesting that psychology ought to take the obvious seriously. What I was saying, essentially, was that the way the tester and the testee experienced and defined the situation should never be assumed to be similar— certainly not identical—and that, by basing interpretations on test item analysis, the psychologist was guaranteeing a very modest level of successful prediction at best and very poor prediction at worst. From today's vantage point, I am puzzled that I did not make it clear that clinical psychology in particular, and psychology in general, was making a major blunder by not studying the differences between problem-solving behavior in contrived-standardized and spontaneous-natural situations. The perception of these differences was already second nature to me, so why did I not come right out and say: "Isn't it time that psychologists start looking at problem-solving behavior outside the test situation? Two factors may have been obstacles to asking this question, factors that still are obstacles to psychologists. The first is that I had not the foggiest notion about how one would study problem solving in nontesting situations; nothing in my training prepared me for studying something over which I had no control and into which I could not intrude. Conceptually and methodologically, I would have been at sea. The second factor was that one of my stocks in trade was standardized testing; it was one of my functions, I got paid to do it, and I knew how to do research with tests and get the studies published. It was as if I was playing to what I knew, not to what I did not know or needed to know. I did what I knew how to do, and part of me stayed away from what I did not know how to do. If I had been able to come right out and say what I was able to say only in later years, it would have meant that I was attacking one of the bases of psychological theory, research, and practice. At that time I had neither the clarity nor the necessary self-confidence (if not arrogance) for such an attack.*

This article was the rationale for the studies of test anxiety that went on for a dozen years or more (Sarason, 1960, 1; 1960, 2). It was also the preliminary statement of my book The Clinical Interaction *(1954, 1). The test anxiety research, which was conventional in conception and methodology, received a lot of attention in different segments of the psychology field.* The Clinical Interaction, *which was less conventional in conception and was critical of certain attitudes toward the use and interpretation of tests (especially projective tests), had little influence, and the book went out of print rather quickly. I am not suggesting that psychology was discernibly poorer because it ignored this book; it was not what I would call a seminal book, if only because it focused on the standardized testing situation. What was important in the book, however, ran counter to what was then the heyday of hell-diving, clinical interpretations. A hell-diving interpretation is one that does not take into account the relationship between content and the clinical interaction. That is very different from an interpretation that may seem farfetched and only distantly related to what a person has said but derives, validly or not, from an assessment of how a person is experiencing the interaction. I used and illustrated this type of clinical interpretation in the culture and personality study conceived by anthropologist Thomas Gladwin (Sarason, 1953, 2).*

3

The Test-Situation and
the Problem of Prediction

I

The purpose of the present paper is to state what seem to be the important determinants of behavior in a testing situation and to examine their implications for the problem of prediction. It should be made very clear at the outset that there is nothing new in the statements of these determinants; nevertheless, they require listing and brief description because the implications to be drawn from them seem to call for a revised approach to the problem of prediction. Attention will be given below to those determinants which are present regardless of the sex, age, and social class of the individual. In addition, there is no intention in the following discussion to convey the impression that the determinants are independent of each other; on the contrary, it is implicitly assumed that they are interdependent variables.

A. The Nature of the Stimulus Materials. The content of the individual's responses, the accompanying expressive behavior, the needs and attitudinal factors engendered are in part a function of the nature of the stimulus materials. How an individual will react to a thematic card cannot be determined from knowing how he reacted to a comprehension item on the Binet.[1] Regardless of the continua (familiarity, physical attributes, shape, etc.) along which one may

S. B. Sarason, "The Test-Situation and the Problem of Prediction," *Journal of Clinical Psychology* 6, no. 4 (October 1950): 378–392. Reprinted with permission.

[1] In the subsequent discussion words like behavior, reactions, or responses refer not only to what an individual says or does but also to the accompanying needs and attitudes which may be overtly manifested or inferred from other behavioral data.

order stimulus materials, the behavior of the individual will in part be a function of that point on a particular continuum that the stimulus material falls.

B. The Nature of the Instructions. An individual who is told that he may respond in whatever way he wants, or that he must complete a task within a certain time limit, or that he must reproduce a stimulus configuration in an exact manner will not necessarily react in a similar fashion to these different instructions.

C. The Purpose of the Testing. How the individual behaves in the testing situation depends on (a) what reasons the psychologist gives for the testing and (b) what the individual has concluded, either before or during testing, are the reasons he is in the particular situation. For example, given three individuals who are alike in several respects, if the first feels that whatever the tests show will "be held against him," he will respond differently from the second who feels that the testing situation is fun, or from the third who looks upon it as downright silliness. The opinion might be ventured here that more than a few psychologists assume that whatever reasons for the testing they have given to the subject are believed and accepted.

D. The Time and Place of Testing. An individual's behavior is a function of when he is being tested and how many times he has experienced the testing situation. What may be equally important is where the individual is being tested: a general hospital, a mental hospital, a school, a psychology laboratory, a private office, or some kind of assessment center.

E. The Psychologist. The behavior of the individual in the testing situation is in part a function of the sex, age, and status of the psychologist. If the purpose of an experiment is either to measure the degree of suggestibility of a subject or to inculcate a feeling of failure, it cannot be assumed that the behavior of the subject will be the same regardless of whether the psychologist is a graduate assistant or a professor in the department.

F. Attitudinal Factors Related to Previous Conditions of Learning. The testing situation engenders varying attitudes toward self and others in different individuals. In some cases feelings of inadequacy, anticipations of failure, and need to avoid anticipated ridicule are aroused even before testing begins. Whatever the needs, attitudes and defenses called forth by the situation, they are a function of previous learning experiences. What one observes in the testing situation is a restricted sample of the ongoing learning process—the content of the sample (i.e., the observed behavior) being a function of past situations which are in some ways similar to the present one. This similarity may be due to several factors among which are the specific stimulus materials and the strength of the previous internal responses. For example, some children whose difficulty in reading is a function of emotional factors may respond less emotionally to the learning of arithmetic; other children may respond with equal involvement to both situations. In the former instance it is as if some kind of discrimination has been made between the two situations, so that the responses elicited by them appear to be rather different; in the latter it is as if a very strong emotional response to one situation has generalized to what objectively appear to be dissimilar stimulus configurations.

II

For the purposes of the present discussion the problem of prediction may be put as follows: from what and to what is one predicting? A common practice is to assign to an individual a score based on his formal test responses and then to predict either his score on another test or his mode of response to another situation. There are several assumptions which usually are made, either explicitly or by inference, when such a procedure is followed, but seldom is there any attempt to evaluate the role and applicability of these assumptions. For example, while the subject's score on the initial test necessarily reflects the variables described in Section I, there is rarely any consideration given to the extent to which each of these variables is either involved or unrelated. If the latter it may be disregarded; if the former it must be taken into consideration if the predictions made are to be based on pertinent variables and not contaminated by the irrelevant ones. A second assumption is that the second situation, regardless of surface similarity or dissimilarity to the first, elicits the same needs and attitudes as did the first situation, a process of generalization of response being facilitated. Since in most studies one does not know or take into account the nature and strength of the variables in the first situation, there is usually little or no evidence for making this second assumption. In those instances where the investigator wishes to predict from one kind of stimulus situation to an obviously different one it is assumed that either the individual will get similar scores because the same kind of behavior is engendered despite the objective differences in the stimulus situations, or that scores will be negatively correlated because of the differences in the stimulus materials. More often than not the scores used in such studies do not reflect the determinants of the behavior but the end product of their interaction.

Three things generally happen to such studies: the results are disappointing and are not reported in the literature; the results are disappointing and are published with the blame directed at the inadequacies of the test; the results are encouraging, which usually means that the correlations are significant above zero; most of the variance is unaccounted for, and prediction to the next case one involves a hazardous procedure.

The point that deserves emphasis is that studies in the prediction of behavior on the basis of psychological tests (or any interpersonal situation) have proved disappointing. It is the contention of the writer that the disappointing results are largely due to the failure to take into account commonly acknowledged significant determinants of behavior, lack of information about the relative importance of these determinants, and the absence of procedures for their measurement. Without knowledge of these determinants one is simply unable to answer the question: from what and to what is one predicting? In the following sections several studies will be discussed in order to concretize some of the points made.

III

Several years ago a study was begun with the aim of discovering how best to predict who will make a good or bad clinical psychologist.[2] Students who had been accepted for graduate work in clinical psychology were assembled in various assessment centers for several days, a wide variety of tests administered to them, "stress interviews" conducted, observations in different kinds of OSS-type of situations made, autobiographies obtained, etc. After these students had been in graduate school for several years they were rated by the staff of the university departments who had contacts with them, and also by the supervisory staff in the field agencies. The predictions made at the time of original assessment proved to be disappointingly poor.

---

[2]This study has not yet appeared in the literature. The present comments are based on a very brief presentation of preliminary findings made by Dr. Lowell Kelley at the Boulder Conference on Graduate Education in Clinical Psychology. What critical comments the writer makes here should not obscure the singular, and perhaps historical, importance of this study in forcing clinical psychology to look very critically at some of its commonly accepted procedures.

The question, of course, is why such poor predictions? There are undoubtedly many factors (unreliability of ratings, for example) which may have contributed to the findings, but attention here will be focussed on the points discussed earlier in the paper.

The first comment that could be made concerns the students' reaction to the stated purpose of the assessment procedure. Although each student knew that he had been accepted for graduate school and had been told that the results of the assessment would in no way affect him, it does not follow that all participants became "ego-involved" to the same degree. Some undoubtedly came to the situation with heightened anxiety and some with little or none. In connection with this it should be pointed out that the assessors were "names" in psychology and experts in the particular procedure they employed. It may be assumed that there was wide variation in the degree and nature of the motivation of the students. In short, individuals probably differed not only in the specific drives or needs engendered but in the degree to which any of these drives was involved. If the kind and level of a drive aroused by a specific stimulus is one of the determinants of the overt response, it is theoretically possible and probable that classification only on the basis of the overt response would be misleading and incomplete. Because two individuals give similar responses to a certain test or respond in an overtly similar manner to a stress situation does not allow one to ascribe their performance to similar psychological factors.

The relevance of several of the other determinants of behavior for the assessment study can be inferred from an examination of the assumption that the various stimulus situations and the ensuing behavior are representative of the situations these students would encounter in graduate school and in field placement. Because a student "went to pieces" in some of the procedures does not mean that attending classes, doing research, administering tests, or doing psychotherapy will evoke similar inadequate behavior. Conversely, the student who never appeared to be perturbed during assessment (perhaps because he knew his future status was in no way at stake?) is not necessarily the one who will sail smoothly through his academic and clinical duties. Aside from the dubious relevance of the criteria, the point should be reiterated that it is only when one knows the "internal" significance of a situation for the individual that one can describe and predict the situations which would elicit similar behavior. Because two children lose their parents at whatever is considered a crucial stage of development obviously does not allow one to say that they were similarly affected by the deprivation. It is not enough to know either the nature of the external stimulus or the content of the individual's formal response. One must also know the kinds of internal behavior (attitudes toward self or others, set, level of anxiety, fantasy content, etc.) with which the overt behavior seems related. It is as important to know the nature of internal as well as external stimuli. Research interest for long has been focussed on the external stimulus and overt behavior with too little attention to devising techniques for getting at and evaluating internal stimuli, studying their relevance for any classification of subjects, and investigating how such data can be reflected in an actuarial statement.

The significance of the assessment study is that it is representative of current thought and practice in clinical psychology. It illustrates how clinical psychologists approach the problem of prediction and how inadequate the approach is. But is would be unfortunate if the major implication drawn from the study is that our present tests are inadequate. Such an implication is in part a justifiable one but to emphasize it would have the result of overlooking our neglect of the determinants of test-situation behavior. In these days of the "total personality," current practice seems inadequate to its assessment.

IV

A concrete clinical example may clarify the previous discussion. There are certain children whose pattern of behavior is sufficiently similar so as to warrant a common label: primary behavior disorder. An abnormal amount of aggressiveness, inability to form satisfactory relationships with people or objects, apparent absence of guilt feelings—these are the characteristics, present since early childhood, which apply to these children and are considered a patterned reaction to unfavorable environmental influences.

A not infrequent experience of therapists with such children is the marked discrepancy between the case history description of behavior and the child's behavior during the initial contacts.

It has been observed frequently that a child with a severe primary behavior disorder is friendliness and sweetness personified during the first few interviews, but thereafter, without fail, returns to the old aggressiveness. Even one of our most experienced and skilled workers felt a question arise in his mind about the correctness of the diagnosis when the boy he was interviewing for the first time was so nice that it seemed impossible to him for this to be the same little devil described in the intake worker's report. However, he soon found out. . . .

It invariably happens that when a child with conduct disorders, a child upon whom all sorts of threats and forms of punishment have been tried unsuccessfully, is finally referred to our agency, the parents have told him that we are going to show him that he cannot go on as he has done, that we are going to be very strict and severe, and so on. Naturally, the child expects unfriendliness, harshness, and threats. To his great surprise, he finds a worker who is quiet and friendly, who is interested in every little thing he mentions. She speaks to him in a civil way and does not scold him. This attitude takes him by surprise and he finds himself disarmed, having no reason or justification for a display of his usual aggressiveness. His hostility finds itself in a vacuum with nothing to fight and the surprising attitude of the worker throws him back into an attitude of friendliness. We have been using the term "surprise reaction" to indicate this behavior: finding to his surprise that there is nothing provoking his hostility, the child reverts, as it were, to the kind of behavior he may have shown before his disorder started. We would be inclined to expect that after the child has had the experience of a pleasant and warm relationship, he might be eager to continue in it, thankful to have found at last a response that he had not met with in a long time, either in his home or in school. But we find ourselves in error very soon and we want to understand what it is that brings about this change.

It would be expected that if one were to predict the behavior of these children on the basis of initial contacts with them, the accuracy of one's predictions would probably be very poor. Unless one viewed the observed behavior in terms of the determinants discussed earlier in this paper, then the child's reactions, present and future, are inexplicable.

V

Lantz's study of "some dynamic aspects of success and failure," while not one specifically concerned with the problem of prediction, illustrates some of the points that have been discussed. The design of the study is briefly given below:

1. 212 nine-year-old boys were studied.
2. They were given 9 items from the Revised Stanford-Binet Scale (L).
3. Each child was put in a ball game situation in which the task was to remove a ball from a box using only one hand. "The ball is to be secured from the box three times in three different ways. Two experiences of success precede the third experience of success or failure and the chosen prize is given only for success on this third problem." Success or failure on the third problem was a function of the subject and not the examiner.
4. The ball game tasks were immediately followed by a comparable set of test items from the Form M scale.

Without going into the details of the analysis it will suffice for the present discussion to state Lantz's conclusion that "The experiences

of success and failure do influence some mental processes more significantly than others. The depressing effect of the experience of failure in decreasing scores is greater than is the exhilarating effect of
success in increasing them."

Since success or failure in the third ball game task was not predetermined by the experimenter but by the subject's performance, the
question arises: why did some boys succeed and others fail in third
task? All the boys appeared to be highly motivated to succeed in
order to win a desired prize. The possibility must be considered that
failure was in some way a function of the kinds of responses engendered by this stressful situation. If such a possibility has merit, then
one must ask if the factors making for a failure performance were
also present in the initial test situation (Form L). The child whose
reactions to the ball game situation had a disorganizing effect on his
performance may also have been the one whose initial Binet performance was also affected by these covert responses. Therefore, it does
not seem justified to assume that performance on the second Binet
testing was being influenced solely by the experience in the ball game
situation. In fact, although Lantz maintains that there was no significant difference between her success and failure groups in the initial
Binet testing, the critical ratio between the means of 2.63 would
indicate otherwise. Even if there was no difference between the two
groups in initial testing, one cannot assume that similar scores stand
in the same relationship to the determinants of behavior in the Binet
situation. If one had a knowledge of these determinants it might well
be that in the case of two individuals with identical scores the prediction might be made that one would fail in the ball game situation
while the other would not.

VI

In his studies of adult intelligence Wechsler found a rather steady
decrease in intelligence test scores beginning at approximately twenty-
five years of age. Wechsler concluded that "the decline of mental
ability with age is part of the general senescent process of the organism
as a whole." This line of reasoning was supported by the similarity
between the curve of mental decline and those of vital capacity and
brain weight. While one cannot doubt the idea of a normal senescent
process, it does not follow that the difference in test scores between
groups of 25 and 50 year old men are solely due to such a process.
When two such groups are viewed in light of what have been called
the determinants of test behavior, it seems reasonable to assume that

the kinds of overt and internal behavior aroused by the test situation are not necessarily the same for the two groups. In a man of 50 the fear of appearing inadequate on an intelligence test might be inordinately strong not only because he *has* slowed up but because he is concerned that he *may* have slowed up. Middle-aged people undoubtedly differ considerably in their need to feel that they are as alert mentally as ever. With a man of 50 many years may have elapsed since he last was in a test situation. The 50 year old man being tested by a much younger person is probably not in the same situation as a 25 year old man being tested by a somewhat older person. In short, one does not know the extent to which differences in scores between such age groups are a function of behavioral factors varying with but not caused by age. Again it would seem that interpretations of findings based on the end product of a highly complicated behavior sequence (anticipatory reactions based on previous learning → external stimulus → internal reactions and drives → articulated response) are theoretically likely to be very incomplete.

VII

The chief conclusion to be drawn from the above considerations is that research in the problem of prediction has neglected important determinants of behavior. One of the reasons for this neglect is probably the failure to view the problem in terms of a systematic theory of behavior. An explicitly stated theory serves at least three very practical purposes: (a) it states publicly what one considers to be the important variables and points the way for experimental verification; (b) it makes the nature of one's disagreements with other researchers more clear and makes resolution of differences by crucial experiments more likely; (c) it makes the inadequacies of the shotgun approach more clear and makes the training of newer generations of students not only easier for the teacher but far more stimulating for the student. Until there are attempts on the level of theory to identify the determinants of behavior, to state the principles by means of which they become related and how they can be measured, putting one's eggs in the basket of "conventional clinical procedures" is not likely to pay off.

Another reason for the neglect of some of the important determinants of behavior is that techniques—observational, physiological, biographical—for evaluating the internal responses to stimulus configurations are either not available or crudely developed. What the subject does not verbalize to the observer (the extent, content, and relevance of his self-verbalizations before and during presentation of the task) is an intervening process which, despite its apparent importance, is very difficult to assess and so has been little studied. Any attempt at theory building must take account of these intervening processes and give impetus to the devising of techniques for their evaluation.

A concluding note: it might be argued by some that the uniqueness of the individual precludes the possibility of predicting his behavior from a knowledge of the behavior of others. In order to predict, the argument runs, one must study *that* individual. It is not the purpose of this paper to examine the implications of this argument for the possibility of establishing a science of behavior. This much might be said in partial answer: if in studying an individual case the psychologist does not start out with a systematic formulation of what are the determinants of behavior, he automatically restricts the kinds of things he will observe, and does not possess a basis for utilizing his wrong predictions as a means of sharpening his handling of the next case he meets. There would be nothing more comforting than to approach the individual case with the knowledge that one's activities have a sound basis in systematic theory and experimental evidence. It may be one would not know what specific weights to give to variables, but at least one would know what the variables are—a situation which does not obtain when we study the individual case today.

BIBLIOGRAPHY

1. Lantz, B. Some dynamic aspects of success and failure. *Psychol. Monogr.*, 1945, *59*, No. 1.
2. (Staff: Jewish Board of Guardians) *Primary behavior disorder in children.* New York: Family Welfare Association of America, 1945.
3. Wechsler, D. *Measurement of adult intelligence.* Baltimore: Williams and Wilkins, 1941, (2nd ed.).

Commentary to Chapter 4

Talking about a community *program for mentally retarded individuals was unusual in 1951. Indeed, although I remembered writing this paper, I thought it was written in the late 1950s, when I had already become aware of the limitations of a purely clinical approach—that is, that a problem exists, or is thought to exist, and* then *the clinician, oriented far more to remediation than to prevention, comes into the picture. The negative consequences of that limitation were compounded by two factors. The clinicians (psychological, medical, educational) who came into contact with mentally retarded individuals were generally uninterested in or uninformed about mental retardation; and the community and certain of its major institutions were unresponsive to the needs of the mentally retarded population. The problems of mentally retarded individuals were understood not in terms of an individual psychology but rather in terms of community values, traditions, and organization, and the goals of prevention (primary, secondary, or tertiary) could not be achieved unless they were conceived in similar terms. Obviously, I was moving out of the confines of clinical psychology and into what was called community psychology a decade later. There was precious little in psychology on which I could depend for conceptual guidance and direction.*

One sentence and one phrase were italicized for emphasis in the original publication. The sentence was "At the present time we spend the large proportion of our time working with problems which never should have been allowed to arise." *I confess that I am proud that the sentence was emphasized, because it signified that I was beginning to question seriously psychology's almost total commitment to the clinical endeavor. It also signified that I was coming to see professionals not as part of a solution but as part of the problem. No less important is that that sentence would not have been written if I were not convinced that the unit of study, for either clinical or preventive purposes, was not the individual but the family in which he or she was an integral part.*

The phrase that was emphasized by italics must be seen in its context:

The emphasis in each case should be on formulating, as soon as possible, a concrete training program and supervising the execution of the program,

even if that means that the clinic comes into the home. When you tell
parents to give their child a particular medication three times a day, the
chances are that this will be done. In the case of the handicapped child,
however, the prescription is a complicated one, not only to understand but
to carry out. Parents need support, encouragement and advice, not only
during the clinic visit, but when they are faced with and responding to
their problems in the natural setting in which they arise.

*Whether assessing problem solving or family behavior, one would be
well advised to observe the natural setting. In suggesting that the
clinic come into the home, I was using the same conceptual rationale
I was to use four years later in the section on problem solving in nontest situations in the Sarason and Gladwin publication (1958, 6).*

*More than any other article I wrote in the 1940s and 1950s, this
one adumbrated the kinds of activities I would later be involved in
and the direction my thinking would take. The culture of schools,
prevention, professional training and professional preciousness, the
inadequacies of an individual psychology, the nature of communities,
institutional change, the creation of new services and settings, the
bureaucratization of human services—facets or hints of each of these
issues are contained in this article. That was the dominant reaction
I had when I reread this article.*

4

Aspects of a Community Program for the Retarded Child

Two weeks ago I received a call from the secretary of a local organized group of parents of cerebral palsied children. It seems that one of the mothers had been trying to get her seven-year-old daughter into the kindergarten of one of the public schools. The school had refused admission because the child was not considered eligible. The mother, believing that the child was eligible, took her for a psychological examination to the out-patient clinic of one of the state training schools. The psychological report was sent to the secretary who was calling me, and who had suggested that the mother have the child given a psychological examination in order to use it as evidence for her belief that the child should be in kindergarten. The psychological report contained the following: (A) a diagnosis was deferred because the child did not talk and the suggestion was made that the child should be seen again when she had learned to talk; (B) on those test items which could be given to the child her mental level seemed to be around three years; (C) the child should not be institutionalized at this time; (D) she should be entered into a kindergarten class if she was considered eligible by the school. The problem with which the secretary of the parent group confronted me was what should she tell the parent?

The above situation is by no means infrequent, and in my own experience is the rule rather than the exception. In trying to understand these frequent situations we might ask this question: How do these situations come about? Before trying to answer this question we first have to ask other questions: What is the nature of the situation here and now? What are the problems with which we should be

S. B. Sarason, "Aspects of a Community Program for the Retarded Child," *The Training School Bulletin* (1952): 201–207.

concerned? Briefly stated, here is what I think are the important aspects of the situation:

1. We are dealing with a parent who has certain beliefs about what her child can learn to do.
2. The mother's beliefs are not shared by school authorities.
3. It is very likely that the mother has a very hostile attitude toward the schools because she feels that they are being unfair and discriminatory.
4. It is also likely that the school authorities consider the mother to be unrealistic and agressive—in short, a nuisance.
5. It is a fact that the schools do not consider this child to be *their* problem.
6. The psychological report does not support the mother's beliefs about the child's capacities.
7. The psychological report contains a recommendation about kindergarten which makes little sense in light of the earlier refusal of the school to admit the child.
8. The psychologist did not discuss his report with the mother.
9. No one, except the local parent group, considered the parent to be their problem, or understood, let alone try to handle, the deep anguish she undoubtedly was experiencing.

Let us now make one assumption: the mother has an unrealistic conception of her child's capacities. If this is so, it is difficult to see how anything done—by the school or the psychologist—was oriented toward helping this mother achieve a more realistic attitude. Telling a mother that her child is not eligible for school may be a valid statement, but in no way does this solve the mother's problem. In fact, making such a statement to a mother is evidence of the fact that the school assumes that only the child is a problem. Telling a mother that her child is not eligible for school without at the same time making concrete proposals concerning the child's training obviously does not help the child, but, just as obviously, increases the severity of the mother's problem. In the case of the psychological examination apparently no attempt was made to convey anything to the mother. The function of a psychological examination is not only to collect data about a child and his problems, but to use these data to help parents react realistically to the child. If the psychologist, for example, had only conveyed to the parent that the child was severely retarded, then he would have been as superficial in his approach to the problem as were the school authorities.

In short, in these situations we are dealing with unhappy, frustrated, conflict-ridden parents who have no one to whom they can turn for help. It is little wonder that they become hostile and direct such feelings toward those who gave them facts but no help. By help

I mean a sustained attempt on the part of some trained person to understand the motivations of the parents, their frustrations and hopes, and by virtue of such understanding, as well as by previous training, enable the parent to accept more realistic and satisfying attitudes. It is worth repeating: in these situations to convey facts should not be taken as synonymous with giving help.

There are other comments one can make about the kind of situation we have been discussing:

1. In most instances, our schools do not understand the psychological ramifications of these situations and it is, therefore, not surprising that they usually do not have the facilities for handling the child or the parent. To handle the situation properly presupposes an understanding of the problems which most educators do not have.
2. The fact that our teacher training schools prepare students in an inadequate way for meeting the problems in this area is but a reflection of an absence of community consciousness about the problem. Too many communities are content to have the handicapped child institutionalized. Too few communities make an attempt to utilize their own facilities or to set up new resources for the handicapped child. I have seen countless children who, after spending several years in an institution, were returned to a community which had little or nothing to offer them in a social, educational or vocational way.
3. The most discouraging feature of these situations is that there usually have been countless earlier opportunities when the parents could have been given a realistic understanding of the problem, prepared for the future problems with which they will be faced, and a concrete program of action formulated. The great bulk of these children have been previously seen by a variety of medical specialists who, for one or another reason, failed to see the social-psychological ramifications for the family, the school and community.

This last point deserves elaboration. There are cases, probably a small minority, where the seriousness of the child's retardation was simply not caught. Sometimes this is due to the incompetence of the physician or psychologist, and sometimes to the fact that our diagnostic methods are not perfect. That our instruments for evaluating intellectual capacity in very young children are not as good as we would like is no reason for not using them. What these imperfections mean is that we must be cautious in assigning weight to a single examination and make provision for a series of examinations with appropriate time intervals. If a series of examinations point to a certain conclusion, we can be more sure of the validity of that conclusion than if it were based on a single examination. One implication of what I have just said is that in the case of very young children the diagnosis should be made by a person with special training in this area. Because a person is a physician or psychologist is no reason for assuming that he has competence in this particular area.

In the great majority of cases, however, the seriousness of the child's retardation was recognized when the child was still very young. If so, one might ask, why does the situation I described earlier arise? There are several reasons:

1. The physician feels that it is not wise to tell the parent until the child is older. The logic behind this unhappy procedure is not always clear. One physician said: "If they can be happy for a few years, why should I stand in their way? They will have enough trouble later on." Some physicians feel that one should not discuss the problem until the parents themselves become aware of it. Whatever the logic the consequences are unfortunate. Ignorance may be bliss, but there are more than a few parents who gladly would have liked to have been spared the bliss. In some cases the awakening is so rude that parents strive (consciously or unconsciously) to prove that the blissful period is not over. They may become hostile to the physician for withholding the information, question his competence, and seek help from others.

2. Frequently the physician does tell the parents about the child's condition, but because he finds this obligation such a painful procedure (it is indeed not a joyous task!) he talks out of both sides of his mouth. At one point he gives glimpses of the true condition, but at another point he reassures the parents with unwarranted optimism. He cannot bring himself to reveal the unvarnished truth which can then serve as a basis for a realistic program for both child and parents. It is to be expected that parents will remember the optimistic and forget the pessimistic aspects of the information which have been conveyed to them.

3. Although the physician may tell the truth to the parents, frequently he fails to relate the educational problems which will confront them in the future with their child. It is easy to tell parents that their child will be able to go to school, but do the parents know that this may mean that the child conceivably might go only as far as the fourth grade? That the schools in the community may not have facilities for their child? That the child may be able only to learn to recognize a few words and do only the simplest of arithmetical tasks? In short, the parents are rarely told what kinds of educational problems they will probably have to face. Unfortunately, too few physicians know the educational system of their community in a way which would allow them to be of more help to parents.

What has all this to do with the setting up of a community program for the mentally retarded? Let me answer this question by giving what I think the aims of such a program should be. First, to detect as early as possible the mentally retarded child; second, to help parents gain a more realistic understanding of their child so that his capacities can be realized; third, to begin to plan with the parent the future program of the child; fourth, to bring our educational system into the picture long before the child is of school age so that the clinic, parent, and school can gain a much better understanding of each other's problems than they now have. In short, the aim of such a program is to prevent personal unhappiness, mutual distrust, self-plaguings, and misdirected use of energies. *At the present time we spend the large proportion of our time working with problems which never should have been allowed to arise.* For example, in the case I described earlier we found a psychologist, a parent, and a school system expending time, effort and money with one result: the parent is probably now more desperate, hostile, confused, and unhappy than before. The point I want to stress is that such an unfortunate situation could have and should have been prevented.

A community program would seem to require the following:

1. A mass educational program the aim of which is to urge parents to bring their children to appropriately staffed clinics for evaluation of their mental and physical growth. The emphasis should be on the preschool child especially those between two and six years of age—ages at which defects become most apparent.
2. The setting up of clinics comprised of medical, psychological and educational specialists. The problems of the handicapped child as well as those of his parents cannot be handled by any one specialist. The emphasis in each case should be on formulating, as soon as possible, a concrete training program and supervising the execution of the program, *even if that means that the clinic comes into the home.* When you tell parents to give their child a particular medication three times a day, the chances are that this will be done. In the case of the handicapped child, however, the prescription is a complicated one, not only to understand but to carry out. Parents need support, encouragement and advice, not only during the clinic visit, but when they are faced with and responding to their problems in the natural setting in which they arise.
3. The community must meet its obligation to provide appropriate educational, occupational and recreational facilities for these children. In providing such facilities attention must be paid to the fact that some day these children will be adults with special problems due to their mental handicaps. The aims of a well-organized program for the childhood and adolescent periods can be defeated by failure to meet the problems of later life.
4. There must be an effort made to get the various professional personnel in this area (a) better acquainted with the need which they should have for each other, (b) the limitations of their own training, and (c) a more keen awareness of the psychological, educational, and community aspects of the problems with which they are dealing.
5. There are many problems in this area for which we do not have the answers. Some of these are medical problems, others are problems in psychological measurement and treatment, while others are concerned with the educational

process. Any program in this area, therefore, must stimulate and support research. If there is any lesson we can learn from the history of science, it is that in the long run research pays off. It is not enough to say we *should* support research in the same way as we say we are for virtue and against sin. We *must* stimulate and support research programs because not to do so guarantees a sterile program, inadequate solutions, and the continued despair of all concerned.

Commentary to
Chapter 5

This paper was prologue to The Creation of Settings and the Future
Societies *(Sarason, 1972, 1). Although the formulation of the creation of settings was not even hinted at in anything I had previously
written, it had been in my thinking, almost obsessionally, for many
years. During the years I was involved in radical politics as a follower
of Trotsky, the central question was why the Russian revolution
failed. Where and why did it go wrong? Why did the dream turn into
a nightmare? Needless to say, the answers I gave were the answers my
political colleagues and leaders gave me, although I was never completely convinced by their explanations. I left the minuscule political
party for a variety of reasons—one of them that I could no longer
parrot slogans and another that I had become both bored and
enamored with destructive organizational intrigue. Reasons for the
failure of the Russian revolution continued to fascinate me, however,
and I would read anything relevant to that question.*

*As luck would have it, my first professional job was in a newly
created state institution for the mentally retarded. I made no connection between the Russian revolution and the Southbury Training
School as instances of the creation of a setting—two or more people
getting together in new and sustained relationships to achieve stated
purposes. (Marriage, legal or otherwise, is the smallest instance; a
revolution to create a new society is the largest instance.) At Southbury I was participating in a new setting, and I worked there long
enough to observe and experience transformations that were antithetical to the initial purposes of the setting. What I learned at
Southbury was that a new setting was not comprehensible by any
psychology I had been taught or had read about. The psychologies
I knew were about individuals who were unrelated to the nature of
the society in which they lived. How the Southbury Training School
was created (that is, why it was created when it was, where it was,
with the structure it had and its embeddedness in government)
could not be understood by any of the existing psychologies. I
came to realize that American psychology was an asocial, ahistorical
psychology by virtue of which the most important substantive
problems of social living went unrecognized or were very incom-
pletely or misleadingly interpreted. Putting it that way, however,*

*makes it seem that my thinking was taking on a clarity that it did not
have. All I feel justified in saying is that I felt I was grappling with an
important problem that I could not formulate. Years later I found
out that one of the obstacles to clarity was that the creation of settings had not been formulated by anyone as a social process and a
conceptual set of issues.*

*The problem did start to get formulated in the context of the
decision in 1961 to start the Yale Psycho-Educational Clinic. There
were many reasons for creating the clinic, but in the early phases of
decision making my interest in the creation of settings was not one
of them. It became the major reason when I found my thinking
going toward whether I would be able to get the clinic going, whether
I was assuming a leadership role for which I might not be adequate.
After all, what did I know about what was involved in creating a setting that I hoped would be a relatively large, multidimensional one?
In the course of these kinds of meanderings, two things happened.
First, the phrase* creation of settings *struck me as a marvelously suc-
cinct description of what I was getting into. Second, and far more
important, that phrase allowed me to see the genotypic similarities
between such phenotypically different instances as the Russian
revolution, the Southbury Training School, and the Yale Psycho-
Educational Clinic. It is hard for me to convey the intellectual
excitement I experienced in interconnecting what I had always
thought were very different phases of my life. Thus, before the
clinic became an organizational and physical reality, I knew that,
for me, the clinic's significance would reside in what I would learn
about the creation of settings.*

*You cannot understand the creation of the clinic unless you see
it in the social context of its time. In the decades that followed
World War II, government (federal, state, and local) took on a degree
of responsibility and initiative unimagined in the pre–World War II
era. It adopted policies that meant that new settings would be
created with fantastic frequency. Those were the days when the
population explosion seemed to be affecting everything and everyone. New schools (each a new setting) could not be built fast enough;
in one community in Connecticut, each new school went on double
sessions from the day it opened. The situation was no different in
higher education, not only in regard to building new colleges and
universities but in terms of myriad new government-supported
training, scholarly, and research settings within the university. In
short, new settings were being created all around us. As the 1960s
became more volatile, the social unrest more evident, the public
and private sectors more sensitive to and fearful of social, genera-*

tional, and racial conflict, a cascade of legislation poured out of legislative halls, and in almost every instance it meant that scores of new settings would be created. I had the opportunity to observe or to consult in many new settings, and I found myself asking, again and again, the Russian revolution question: "Why is this setting falling apart, or why is this setting so inconsistent with its original purposes?" That was only the tip of the iceberg, however, because what I learned was that many, perhaps most, settings never get to the point of operation. They die before they should come into this world. Conceptually, these aborted efforts are as important as those that become operational.

Although the book The Creation of Settings and the Future Societies *has more scope and contains far more detail than this article, the guts of the formulation of the problem are here. I never expected that the book would receive much response or that it would be in print a decade after it was published. The book has more of an audience outside psychology than inside, and I explain this largely on the basis that so much of psychology focuses on the individual organism and ignores the ways in which the nature and traditions of the social order impinge on the settings of which each of us is a part. This criticism of American psychology is discussed in my 1981 book* Psychology Misdirected: The Psychologist in the Social Order. *When I reread the article that follows, I was amazed to find that two of its pages contain the core idea of the later book, almost word for word.*

From the vantage point of the passing years, I can see that this article was a switching point in my personal, intellectual, and professional developement. In this article I gained the security to write without worrying about what those who preceded me said. I knew I was breaking new ground, but, although that was intimidating, it did not stop me from being forthright about the importance I attached to what I was saying. I was criticizing the Achilles heel of American psychology; I was departing from traditional problem areas in psychology; and I did not care what the consequences might be.

Let me clarify this by pointing out again that this collection of papers contains nothing from the twelve years of the Test Anxiety Project, the series of research studies that made me visible in American psychology. By conventional standards it was a very successful project, and then as now I considered its contributions very respectable. In substance and methodology, however, it was very conventional research and contributed little to my intellectual development. Indeed, as will become clear in later pages, this project was so successful that it delayed my moving in new directions. I was a victim of success, an example of oversocialization into main-stream psychology. Recognition of what had happened to me was one of the factors that led me to the creation of the Yale Psycho-Educational Clinic and served to embolden me to start thinking about the limitations of American psychology—to start taking distance from my own field, to ask what was not being studied, and to return to my real interest, the nature of American society and psychology's place in it. Divesting myself of the Test Anxiety Project radically changed my view of myself and of psychology. Given the consequences, I suppose I should be grateful for that project. The phrase creation of settings, *with the emphasis on* creation, *pinpoints what was bothering me at the time.*

5

The Creation of Settings:
A Preliminary Statement

This chapter is an initial attempt to raise and briefly discuss two questions. How do people go about creating new settings? (I am using the terms settings, programs, organizations, institutions interchangeably.) What body of theory and practice is available as guidelines for those who have the responsibility of creating settings? Although I am discussing these questions within the narrow context of certain aspects of the mental health fields, it is my hope in later publications to demonstrate the generality of the problem in as phenotypically diverse activities as art, research and industry, as well as in social-political movements which have as an aim the creation of new institutions. The American Constitutional Convention, the Russian Revolution, a new business, a new university, a new hospital or clinic, the behavior of researchers—despite the obvious and many ways in which these events and activities differ, they involve the human mind in the production of end projects which will be consistent with original purposes. That is to say, these end products are supposed to have a meaning and structure which are not defeating of the purposes of the creators or the interests of those for whom the end products were developed. When in his pioneering book in 1860 on the Italian Renaissance Burckhardt (4) entitles the first chapter "The State as a Work of Art"—meaning that it is the product of processes "of reflection and calculation"—he was, I think, recognizing that the creation of

S. B. Sarason, "The Creation of Settings: A Preliminary Statement," *Social Psychiatry* 47 (1969). Copyright © 1969, The Association for Research in Nervous and Mental Diseases. Reprinted with permission.

settings has kinship with many other types of important human activity from which we have much to learn.

When one looks over the history of the mental health fields one sees time and again how they have changed—in practices, research and training—as a function of a new conception, theory or technique. Shock, drugs, lobotomy, psychoanalytic theory, group techniques, nondirective therapy, ink blots and existentialism are but a few examples of this generalization. In the past decade, however, a new "problem" has begun to influence markedly and fatefully the mental health fields, a problem which does not reflect a new technique or even a new idea but rather the guilt-laden discovery of a population with which our fields have had in the past only a peripheral relationship. I refer, of course, to the so-called poverty population. There was precious little in our theories, and even less in our techniques, to justify any optimism that we would have much to contribute (7). It was in the nature of the problem, precisely because it reflected something seriously wrong with our social order, that the pace and direction of change would be taken out of our hands and would be determined by government policy and instrumentalities. When federal policy is buttressed by money, the processes of change, for good and for bad, are started. My aim in this chapter is 2-fold: to examine some of the consequences of these changes, and then to state a problem, the creation of settings, that I consider to be the crucial one with which our fields will have to grapple over the coming decades. I fully realize the two dangers involved in such a discussion: one of them stems from any attempt to attain perspective on the present, and the other inheres in any attempt to read the future.

THE PSYCHOLOGY OF THE INDIVIDUAL

In a basic sense the mental health fields have rested on a psychology of the individual, i.e., the thinking, theories and practices of the mental health worker are primarily concerned with the behavior of individuals and how such behavior may be modified. The most obvious manifestation of this is in the word "patient." The private practitioner, the clinic, the hospital think in terms of numbers of patients. One has only to peruse our professional journals to conclude that most workers spend much of their time thinking about what goes on inside individuals. It would indeed be surprising if the situation were otherwise, in light of the modal training program in which theorizing about and working with individuals occupy most of the trainee's time. The clinical tradition (in contrast, for example, to the public health tradition) is one in which the individual is made the focus of attention and the primary object of responsibility.

What implications may be drawn from the fact that our university centers and professional societies, as well as individual professionals, belatedly recognize or feel a responsibility to engage in different ways in programs developed for the poverty population? There are many implications, but several are more important than others for my present purposes. The first implication is that there was relative unawareness in the mental health fields that they occupied a certain place in the social order and that their place in the social order inevitably affected and reflected the outlook and values of those in these fields. Put in another way, if in a field there is general unawareness of the obvious fact that it is embedded in a social structure—that society is not a random, ahistorical, static collection of individuals, groups and classes—the possibility is maximized that the thinking and practices of those in the field will be parochial and that this parochialism will be surrounded by beliefs that act as impermeable barriers to "foreigners and foreign ideas." As a consequence, it takes a major upheaval in the social order, such as a war, an economic depression or a race riot, to confront individuals in professional fields with their parochialism and with the need to change or elaborate their practices, values and theories.

The second implication is an amplification of something embedded in the first one, i.e., that the psychological theories that dominated, and still dominate, the mental health fields simply did not address themselves to the nature of our society. Put in another way, the theories were not, other than in a superficial manner, social-psychological in nature. Furthermore, the psychological theories were developed and presented as if they were independent of the relation of the theoriest to the social structure. The genius of Einstein resided in his demonstration that the position of the observer in relation to events was a problem with which a theory concerning those events had to deal explicitly. Psychological theorists seem unwittingly to have assumed that the statements that they make about human behavior are independent of the place or position that they occupy in the social order.

A qualifying point is necessary here. There have been numerous attempts, many of them productive, to bring together psychological theories on the one hand with sociological and anthropological data and conceptions on the other hand. Most of these attempts to arrange a healthy marriage have come from those outside the mental health fields.[1] This may account for my impression that the social scientist approached the marriage with far less ambivalence than did the mental health workers. The social scientist seemed to know in a gut kind of way that the mental health fields had ideas and knowledge which could make the union a truly fruitful one. The mental health fields contemplated the union with much less eagerness and optimism. They viewed it in two ways: as a trial marriage which possibly could last, or as a luxury rather than as a necessity; neither view would be considered by a marriage counselor as portending happiness.

What the mental health fields did not realize—what their existing theories could not direct them to see—was that in entering the union they were housing a time bomb in the sense that the amalgamation of psychological and social science theory could not fail, sooner or later, to direct attention to the relation between psychological theories and mental health practices. It happened sooner rather than later because that is the kind of world we are living in. Mental health practices did have a basis in theory, i.e., they were based on assumptions about what people are, how they get that way and the conditions in which they change and can be helped to change.

When the time bomb exploded, and there are still some who have neither seen or heard it, several things became clear. First, mental health practices were not as effective as anyone would like them to be. Second, mental health workers spent a lot of time with relatively few individuals who were representative of only certain parts of our social structure. Third, it was indisputably true that neither now nor in the foreseeable future could mental health workers be trained in quantity sufficient even to begin to meet the problems of *individuals*. Fourth, aside from the techniques involved in working with individuals and small groups, psychological theories were dishearteningly sterile

---

[1] Although this is true of the majority of these attempts, I am of the opinion that the most important of them have come from within the mental health fields. I refer specifically to the writings of Kardiner, Sullivan, Erickson and Fromm. However, it is important to note that of these four only Fromm has explicitly addressed himself to two important issues: the relation between the theories and practices of the mental health fields and their place in our social order, and the inadequacies of these theories and practices in conceptualizing and dealing with conditions making for disordered lives and living. It is my impression that it is precisely because Fromm has talked to these issues that he tends to be viewed as an outsider (trainees in our university centers are not required to read Fromm with anywhere near the frequency with which they are asked to read the others) in much the same way that Freud was regarded in his early years by medicine, psychology and the social sciences. Some of our more orthodox colleagues seem to have difficulty in comprehending that Fromm's critique should not be viewed as polemical or philosophical but rather as a necessary consequence of his theoretical position on the nature of man *and* society. Far more than anyone else on the current scene Fromm possess the "sociological imagination" so beautifully described and discussed by C. Wright Mills (6).

in developing new kinds of service. Fifth, and perhaps most important and fateful—and you will excuse me if I state it the way that I ordinarily think it—the craziness of people in a very important way reflects the craziness of the settings or systems of organizations in which they have been or currently are involved. We know this about the setting which we call a family, but that is only one of many settings contributing to craziness, i.e., to inadequate, self-defeating, self-limiting, other-destroying behavior.[2] The concepts of setting, the relationships among settings and the relationships of these concepts to those of social class and social structure—these are the kinds of concepts and relationships that psychological theories must assimilate, and this process is going on. The focal point of resistance to this process is not primarily on a conceptual or theoretical level but on the plane of its significance for practices and training.

I indicated at the outset that one cannot understand the current turmoil in the mental health fields without taking account of the so-called War on Poverty. In essence, when the government said (and this includes a number of mental health workers who had a clear conception of what was wrong but a not so clear conception of what should be done) that it could no longer countenance the consequences of the unequal availability of health services, it was not only stating a moral challenge to the health professions but also facing them with the necessity of developing new conceptions and practices. Anyone who has any familiarity with our university training centers is well aware of the conflicts engendered by government policies and the monies available to implement them. The conflicts on a manifest level concern what one should do, but the more serious conflict concerns how one should think, i.e., the development of new and more broad conceptualizations from which new strategies for training and practice may flow.

My purpose here has been not to prove but rather to state the following points.

1. The mental health fields have been dominated both in theory and practice by what I have termed a psychology of the individual.

2. Theories and practices have been presented and described as if

---

[2] It is a frequent source of surprise to us to learn that many mental health workers have difficulty grasping the idea that behavior is (among other things) inevitably a reflection of characteristics of settings. They know this about the setting that we call a family, but they have difficulty transferring the principle to other settings which are fateful to how lives are lived. It is second nature for mental health workers to think about the individual and his family (a way of thinking which has foundations in theory and practice) although it is far from second nature to think similarly about the individuals in other contexts. This reflects the narrowness of the theories used, a narrowness which can be lethal for the development of new practices in new settings.

they did not themselves reflect the social order in which they were developed.[3]

3. Social processes have brought to the fore problems that demonstrate not only the second point but also the unpreparedness of the mental health fields to deal with these problems on the levels of theory, practice and training.

4. These societal problems have lent a sense of urgency to the union of psychological and social science theory at the same time that this union is creating a major identity crisis in the mental health fields.

Elsewhere (8) some colleagues and I have described in some detail our efforts at the Yale Psycho-Educational Clinic to take seriously the points raised in the present chapter. What I would like to do now is to state a problem that we have come upon and that illustrates in an unusually clear way two things: the inadequacies of existing psychology theory and the intellectual constrictions imposed on the clinician who, by virtue of being a clinician, comes into action only when a problem has already developed, be it a problem of the individual, a group or a setting. One may not enjoy the analogy, but I think that the mental health worker can be characterized as a psychological fireman who, in a vast forest, spends his time putting out brush fires, hoping that they are really put out, not knowing where the next fire will erupt, secure only in the knowledge that other firemen in the forest are having the same experiences and degree of success, and disquieted by the nagging thought that there must be a way of tending to a forest by means of which the possibility of fires is discernibly reduced. But if the psychological fireman spends most, if not all, of his time putting out fires, the cathecting of nagging thoughts is really asking for too much. But I must first apologize to the real firemen because they do spend time in efforts which make fires less likely to occur.

---

[3]Theories and practices will always reflect the social order in which they are developed. My point is that the recognition of this point in theory building forces one to face issues of social change, i.e., to anticipate, in broad outline at least, how the social order will (or may) change and the consequences for practice. This is, of course, the case in political and economic theory. For example, a case in point is the central concern of many social scientists with the present and future pattern of relationships between the social order and technological advances. Heilbronner's recent book *The Limits Of American Capitalism* (5) is, in my opinion, an excellent example of how, on the basis of an analysis of aspects of the existing social order, one can begin to examine what the future social order may be. Although his is primarily an economic analysis, the social-psychological implications of his analysis are many and profound, both for social-psychological theory and for mental health practices.

THE CREATION OF SETTINGS

I am quite sure that I am not far wrong when I say that in the past two decades more new settings have been created than in the entire previous history of the human race. For example, when the Project Head Start legislation was implemented it meant that several thousand discrete settings were to be created, i.e., in each setting a group of people (children and adults) were to be brought together in sustained relationships to meet certain objectives. When one considers that Project Head Start is but one of thousands of federal programs, in addition to those created by states, communities, industry, etc., it is clear that we are dealing with a fantastic rate of creation of settings. In addition, one must keep in mind that within our larger institutions and organizations (e.g., hospitals, schools, universities) new programs are constantly being implemented, programs which result in grouping or regrouping of individuals into new and presumably enduring relationships for the attainment of stated objectives. If I am at all correct about the frequency of setting creation or program implementation, it must have important implications for (or be a significant reflection of) the social structure of our society as well as for understanding the lives of people; but these are not issues that I am able to take up here.

And now to relate this to what I have said earlier in this chapter. Because of the necessity to be brief, let me establish the relationship by stating what I consider to be two facts and then posing a question:

1. In recognizing that the needs of society would not be met by relying predominantly on psychotherapeutic techniques, an increasing number of mental health workers now spend time in studying and evaluating various kinds of settings. It is probably the case, although we have no evidence on this, that the consultant focuses far less on the needs or problems of individuals in the setting than on problems which reflect malfunctions in the setting or system. From the standpoint of role models, the mental health consultant is very similar to the industrial psychologist who views the presenting problem as a reflection of the system. More important than role models is the fact that the mental health consultant, like the industrial psychologist, tends to deal with what I have called the craziness of systems and settings (1–3).

2. It seems already that the demand for mental health consultants will far exceed the supply, now and in the foreseeable future. It is very likely that this discrepancy, as in the case of the demand-supply relationship in psychotherapy and psychoanalysis, will widen as time goes on if only because of the rate at which settings are being created.

3. In light of the rate at which settings are created, taken together with the discouragingly frequent tendency for settings adversely to affect behavior and to generate interpersonal problems which defeat or dilute the purposes of the setting so as to require the assistance of the outside consultant, one has to ask: should we not direct our attention to how one can create settings so as to minimize craziness and the need for outside consultants (who usually will not be available)?

In our recent book (8) we describe in detail our consultant role in various community settings, and it was as a result of these experiences that we found ourselves dealing with problems which in large measure reflected, among other things, characteristics of the settings. That is to say, we were dealing with problems generated by a whole host of interrelated system characteristics: formal and informal relationships, explicit and implicit uses of power, vehicles for and qualities of communication, the relationship of individuals to planning, perception of goals and history, etc. There must, we thought, be another way of creating settings which would not generate so much self- and setting-defeating behavior. We were not comforted by the thought that our experience indicated that settings organized, developed and administered by mental health workers contained as many self-defeating system characteristics as those settings to which mental health workers served as consultants. This should not be taken as an *argumentum ad hominem*, so to speak, but as a suggestion that expanded awareness of ourselves in our own settings may make us better observers of and interveners in the settings which we are called upon to improve.

The first question we asked was: faced with the task of creating a setting, particularly one devoted to human service, what theory and experience are available as guidelines? The answer, unfortunately, is very clear. Existing psychological theories, be they primarily individual or social-psychological in nature or emphasis, do not address themselves to the problem of the creation of settings. There is an ever growing body of theory and observation on "sick" settings—which in a few years will probably be equal in bulk to that of "sick" individuals—but little or nothing on the creation of healthy settings. The problem will not be clarified because of the tendency, understandable in clinicians, to focus on, or to be called to treat, the malfunctioning setting. Freud, fortunately, understood well that the picture of early childhood gained from the analysis of neurotic adults should not be confused with the picture that one would obtain from a direct study of origins. In relation to the present problem one must hope that we will be ever aware that our existing theory and knowledge about organizations and institutions primarily reflect experience with chronologically mature, malfunctioning settings; this can mislead us as to how such malfunctioning developed but, more important, I think, it does appear to be very helpful to someone who wants to create, or has to create, a new setting.

The lack of guidelines forced us to another question: how do people go about creating settings? In light of the lack of relevant theory and description, a number of us at the Psycho-Educational Clinic have taken advantage of several opportunities to observe and participate in the process. The first opportunity is very partially described in our book (8). The second, and a far more significant and sophisticated attempt, involved Dr. Ira Goldenberg's assuming the responsibility for organizing and developing a Residential Youth Center for inner city boys between the ages of 16 and 21. The third opportunity, involving Dr. Francis Kaplan, George Zitnay and myself, is very recent and concerns an institution which will not be a physical reality for at least 2 years.

Obviously, it will be some time before we will be able to organize and present our thoughts, experiences and data in coherent form, but certain general statements can already be made.

1. In creating a setting the person or persons with responsibility quickly became overwhelmed by two strong, related feelings: that the problem was far more difficult than they imagined, and that they had no explicit guidelines for determining what they would do, the sequence in which it might be done, how to anticipate problems, etc.[4] This becomes most revealing when the person or persons with responsibility are professional individuals with a demonstrated competence in dealing with the dyadic or small group therapeutic situation. In the therapeutic situation they are relatively at ease. They have a feeling of security about what they are doing, why they are doing it and how it is likely to come out. They have wedded theory with technology which, despite its shortcomings, serves as a psychological map. Faced with the task of creating a setting they tend to feel as if they were alone in a small boat on uncharted seas, with a cloud cover obscuring the stars, possessing no reliable compass—and worried lest the frail boat spring a leak. The regressive aspect of the last part of this metaphor does not require that I say anything about anxiety in the creation of settings.

2. In our society, at least, creating a setting involves one with a

---

[4] This probably is not always the case, particularly when those with responsibility approach the task in a predetermined, "businesslike" way, armed with organizational charts which prevent the anticipation and recognition of substantive problems. The generalizations offered above hold, in our experience, for those individuals with acute awareness that the relation between an organizational chart and the actual functioning of a setting may be like that between an individual's *curriculum vitae* and the "real individual."

variety of existing settings which may have different purposes and traditions but with which one must develop and maintain relationships. One comes quickly to recognize that (as in the case of a modern nation) the problems of coordinating them in a non-self-defeating way are enormous.

3. At every step of the process, and particularly in the earliest stages when relatively few people are involved, every decision or action tends to have immediate consequences for the group. My point does not concern goodness or badness of action or decision. What I wish to emphasize is that decisions and actions have consequences for relationships within the small group and, since in the earliest stages the small group tends to consist of those in important positions, unawareness of this fact, or not having built-in vehicles for ensuring awareness of it, can engender a pattern or style of talking and relating which over time results in full blown organizational craziness. (The only good argument I can come up with against the use of the term craziness is that what we call craziness seems to be the norm for organizations.)

4. In the earliest stages, as we indicated, there is usually a small group of individuals involved; this is practically always the case when a physical structure has to be built to house the setting. The point at which this small group begins to enlarge, and this enlargement may involve one or more newcomers, is always a danger point because it involves the old and the new, the insider and outsider, those who have belonged and those who want to belong, those who have had power in some form or other and those who will want power. When this enlargement takes place very rapidly, and again *when there are no built-in vehicles for anticipating, recognizing and handling the problem*, the setting tends quickly to become a highly differentiated one in which the parts are maladaptively related and *the overall purposes of the setting become secondary to the purposes of its component parts*.

5. Creating a setting is, from a purely intellectual point of view, a fantastically complicated array of problems. In fact, this conceptual complexity is of such a high order that, when its magnitude is recognized by those whose responsibility it is to create a setting, it results in strengthening the tendency to simplify the problem. The need to simplify problems as a defensive tactic to protect the self is inversely related to the degree of awareness of the complexity of the issues and its consequences. This is identical in principle to the situation of the artist who knows what he wants to create but is faced with the knowledge that he cannot, or will not be able to, do it. In both instances the consequences can be disastrous for the individual and his products.

6. There is an ego-syntonic expectation that there will be a time in the history of the setting when there will be fewer problems (within the setting and between settings) so that those who created the setting can look forward to a reduction in the level of intellectual and emotional turmoil required by the need for vigilance and the anticipation, recognition and handling of problems. It is identical to the myth entertained by most people entering therapy or analysis, i.e., that when it is all over they will be free of conflict and anxiety, competent to handle any or all problems. In the case of the creators of settings, the awareness that the myth is a myth can wittingly or unwittingly set into motion a way of viewing and relating to the setting so that the level of struggle is indeed reduced at the same time that the level of craziness in the setting increases—one produces what one wanted to avoid.

These generalizations (highly selective) may or may not be well stated, and it may be that we or others will find out over time that, as is usually the case, understanding the interrelationships among issues and processes is less likely to result in conceptual distortion than becoming enamored of one or another aspect of the complexity. The two purposes for stating these generalizations were to indicate the degree of complexity with which we are dealing and to suggest that the craziness of settings may have its roots in the earliest stages of their development.

The creation of settings is not a problem contained in or derivable from existing psychological or social science theory. I am of the belief that it may well be *the* problem the recognition of which will facilitate the development of that kind of heightened consciousness or awareness which will lead to conceptions that will both encompass and transform existing theories of man *and* society. The transformation will result in conceptions of man *in* society. If such a transformation begins to take place—which is but another way of saying that our styles and categories of thinking will have begun to change—one may look forward to the day when those in our fields of inquiry and practice will look with understanding, condescension and amusement at our current tendencies to win battles and lose wars, to react instead of act, to engage primarily in works of repair instead of works of creation and worst of all, to fail to see, and hence to take measures to correct, the crucial problem: i.e., that our theories and practices were the inevitable consequences of our times, society and history. Freud taught us a good deal about why we had to take distance both from ourselves and from the patient. The next difficult task is to reach that higher elevation which may enable us to catch insightful glimpses of the interrelationships among ourselves, our theories, practices and society. But to strive for the higher elevation implies (as it does in the act of seeking personal therapy) that we have made the crucial decision that movement and change are necessary.

REFERENCES

1. Argyris, C.: Interpersonal Competence and Organization Effectiveness. Richard D. Irwin, Inc., Homewood, Ill., 1962.
2. Argyris, C.: Organization and Innovation. Richard D. Irwin, Inc., Homewood, Ill., 1965.
3. Argyris, C.: How effective is the state department? Yale Alumni Magazine, 1967, May, 38–41.
4. Burckhardt, J.: The Civilization of the Renaissance in Italy. Phardon Publishers, Greenwich, Conn.
5. Heilbronner, R. L.: The Limits of American Capitalism. Harper & Row, Publishers, Inc., New York, 1966.
6. Mills, C. W.: The Sociological Imagination. Grove Press, Inc., New York, 1961.
7. Sarason, S. B.: Towards a psychology of change and innovation. Am. Psychologist, *22*:227–233, 1967.
8. Sarason, S. B., Levine, M., Goldenberg, I. I., Cherlin, D., and Bennett, E.: Psychology in Community Settings: Clinical, Vocational, Educational, Social Aspects. John Wiley & Sons, Inc., New York, 1966.

Commentary to
Chapter 6

We are carriers of history just as we are carriers of genes, and in both cases we are rarely aware in our daily lives that we are carriers. We cannot see genes, just as we cannot see history. However unsophisticated people may be about genetic processes and transmission, they are even more so when it concerns how they carry history. We know that we were begotten and that we may similarly beget, but very few people know how their present is the offspring of an alive past and how that present may spawn different futures. Societies differ dramatically in terms of how their members see themselves as points in a continuous stream of history, as conduits through which history flows. On one extreme, the members of a society may draw no sharp distinction between present and past; the present is the past in a new guise, just as the present will be transformed into a future. On another extreme—and our society should be placed near that extreme—the present tends to be sharply demarcated from the past. The past is a museum of relics, not a linking part of the present. It was not by chance that it was in Western society that methods such as psychoanalysis were invented to allow an individual to rediscover the past in the present. These methods are testimony to the strength of our internal obstacles to remembering and identifying with a personal *past. These obstacles are not understandable only in individual terms but also must be seen in relation to the supports they receive from the dominant features of the society. If remembering and identifying with a personal past are not easy, it should not be at all surprising if remembering and identifying with a societal past would be even more difficult.*

American psychology has walked a not-so-fine line between ahistoricism and antihistoricism. Enamored as it has been of the individual organism, psychology appears to embrace individual history, but what an amazingly narrow view of history it has been! Individual history has been treated as unrelated to social history, racial and ethnic history, intellectual history, and political-economic history. Read any *case history illustrating* any *psychological theory and you will understand what Murray Levine meant by his felicitous phrase "intrapsychic supremacy" and what C. Wright Mills (1959) meant by "psychologisms": inappropriately trying to explain social move-*

ments and social-historical forces with concepts derived from individual psychology.

The nature-nuture controversy of the early 1970s was the latest of several controversies that have erupted in our society. This one was no less ahistorical in substance than earlier ones. That the proponents of nature would downplay social-cultural history was not surprising, but I was surprised that the advocates of nurture gave only token recognition to how individual and social history were inextricably related. This should not have surprised me, because American social science in general, and psychology in particular, have never really confronted the issue of how individual history contains social-cultural history. More specifically, they have not come to terms with the issues formulated so well in 1935 by John Dollard in The Criteria for the Life History. On the surface, Dollard's book says nothing about the nature-nurture controversy, but from the first time I read it I knew that his formulations raised questions that had to be answered before one could begin to assign weights to nature and nurture. That is also why I was both delighted and excited when I first read the social-historical chapters John Doris wrote for our book Psychological Problems in Mental Deficiency (1969, 2). If the participants in the nature-nurture controversy had read Dollard's and Doris's writings, the controversy might have had some productive consequences.

REFERENCES

Dollard, J. *Criteria for the life history*. New Haven: Yale University Press, 1935.
Mills, C. W. *The sociological imagination*. New York: Oxford University Press, 1959.

6

Jewishness, Blackishness, and the Nature-Nurture Controversy

Those who have participated in the recent version of the nature-nurture controversy have, for the most part, neglected to confront the derivation of their time perspective in relation to social change in general and historically rooted group attitudes and performance in particular. As in past versions of the controversy, the issues have centered around personal and social values, methodology, the content of the measuring instruments, sampling problems, and genetic theories and laws, and the consequences of these issues for programs of social action. There seems to be recognition by all that social history is an important variable, that inequity and prejudice have been and are rampant, and that it is probably impossible at the present time to discuss the controversy in a dispassionate way. Within scientific circles it is an explosive issue, just as it is in the society at large. I assume that if a study were done asking people if they thought that future versions of controversy (say 20 or 40 years from now) would be conducted in a less explosive climate, almost all would reply in the negative. Indeed, many would probably predict a more explosive climate. If a similar study had been done 50 years ago when, after World War I, the nature-nuture controversy was once again peaking, far fewer people would have correctly predicted the present climate of social explosiveness in which the controversy is taking place. (At that time, interestingly enough, blacks were not central to the controversy. The inferiority of blacks was not then a burning issue, presumably because it was uncritically accepted by most people [white and black] as a fact which did not need to be labored. It was the flood of immi-

S. B. Sarason, "Jewishness, Blackishness, and the Nature-Nurture Controversy," *American Psychologist* 28, no. 11 (November 1973): 962–971. Copyright 1973 by the American Psychological Association. Reprinted by permission.

grant groups from Europe and Asia that brought together questions of national policy and the status of knowledge about the determinants of intellectual performance.) Today, sides have been taken and with a degree of partisanship that the passage of time will not easily change— a variant of my thesis that changes in attitude and performance of historically rooted groups are relatively immune to change except when viewed from a time perspective in which the basic measuring unit may be a century. When I say a century I do not mean it in a precise or literal way, but rather as a means to emphasize a time perspective far longer than that which we ordinarily adopt.

For a statement and description of my position convincingly to reflect my thinking requires that I be unusually personal and relatively unhindered by considerations of modesty, politeness, and that undefined criterion of "good taste." I shall talk about aspects of myself and my family not only because they are the "data" I know best, but because I assume (phenomenologically I *know*) that I am quite representative of Jews, possessed of all the ingredients that comprise Jewishness. What I have to say has been said, and far better, by other Jews. I justify going over old ground because, as the title of this article suggests, I wish to relate it to an important and fateful social and scientific issue. Here, too, I make no claim to originality, although I believe that I provide an emphasis that has been lacking in the scientific literature.

JEWISHNESS

I begin with my father, a simple, unassuming, relatively inarticulate man who spent a long working life as a cutter of children's dresses. He was not an impressive person. He did not read books, but he went to synagogue and obviously knew the Old Testament (in Hebrew) backward and forward. As he prayed, he kept the books open and turned the pages, but rarely did more than glance at them. He recited the prayers in a most undeviating, ritualistic manner. Beginning at age 8 or 9, having enrolled me in Hebrew school, he expected me to sit and pray with him. Of course, I did not understand what I was reading (or even why), and when from time to time my boredom and anger forced me to ask why the book could not be put into English, he never deemed the question worthy of a response.

He loved children and had a gentleness with them to which they responded, but my memory contains nothing that would support the notion that he had other than a primitive notion of children and learning. The early sources of my anger toward my father were many, but two are particularly relevant here. One concerns a leather-covered Oxford dictionary which I had not the strength to pick up until I was six or seven. I still have the dictionary, and when it comes to its weight I know whereof I speak. I never saw my father use that dictionary, and to me its presence was symbolic of his selfishness: Why did we have *that* around the house when we (I) needed other things? Why didn't we hide it, sell it, or throw it out? Occasionally I would peruse its pages, but the book was so large and heavy that even when I did not have to hold it, I could not comfortably use it. Related to this was our battle about the *New York Times*, which he bought and read every day. Why buy a newspaper that did not have funnies? How more selfish could a father be than to deprive his children of newspaper funnies, particularly on Sundays when all other newspapers contained loads of them? I hated the *New York Times*, which, I need not tell you, I now read every day. I also have an aversion to funnies and truly cannot comprehend why my wife and daughter read them first when the local paper arrives—and sometimes even argue about who will read them first.

And then there were my older male cousins who, when I was in elementary school, were preparing to go to college. At that time I knew as much about college as I did about astronomy. There was a place called college and there were stars in the sky, and that exhausted my knowledge of both. But in the numerous meetings of the extended family that word *college* kept coming up in reverent and awesome tones. Cousin Leo was not going to any college, he was going to a place called Cornell and that showed (not to me) that Leo was smart because not many Jewish boys were *allowed* there. And if Leo did well there, as *of course* he would, he was then going to go to still another kind of college and become a doctor. Cousin Moey was a very smart fellow, too, and wasn't it too bad that he had to work during the day and go to college at night. Go to college at night! What kind of craziness was that? To me that meant he couldn't listen to the radio at night, those being the days when having a radio was still a novelty. It was during these early years that I kept hearing the phrase "He will make something of himself" applied to some of my relatives.

There was also Leo's brother, Oscar, who was special. If I had available to me then the words I have now I would have described Oscar to my friends as smart-smart. That's the way the family regarded him. But Oscar posed a real problem because he played football, and extremely well. He was as good in football as he was in the classroom. That Oscar was on the small side was only one reason for family opposition to playing football. It was important because he might get "good and hurt," not able to go to school, and maybe not even go to college. The more important point was that nice Jewish boys, particularly if they were smart-smart, didn't play football. That was for the gentiles (goys), who were by nature not smart; they were, instead, and again by nature, crudely physical and aggressive. Football was quintessentially goyish, and it was stupid for Jewish boys to compete in that arena. David may have slain Goliath, thanks to God, but that was in another world. Let's respect David, but let us not go so far as to identify with his actions! One Saturday morning I walked into my cousin's apartment—we lived upstairs, those being the days of extended families in restricted areas, and I use the word "restricted" in its geographical and discriminatory senses—and I heard my aunt yelling and screaming in Oscar's room. There was Oscar curled up womblike being pounded by my aunt at the same time that she was telling him and the world what she thought of a Jewish boy who was going to play football for his high school *on Saturday*. What had she done to deserve such punishment? What would *they* think? "They" referred to all her Jewish friends and neighbors who, she was sure, would both blame and sympathize with her on one of the worst fates a Jewish mother could experience. How could a mother stand by and watch her child, with such a "good head," go straight to hell? It was an awesome display of physical energy and verbal imagery— my Aunt Jennie was regarded by all as having no equal when it came to using and inventing the Yiddish equivalents of longshoreman language. When her physical energy was spent (the verbal flow never ceased), Oscar got up from the bed, collected his football suit, calmly but sweetly said good-bye, and went off to join the goyim in defense of the glory of Newark's Barringer High School. Needless to say, when he went to Brown, where he was quite a football player during the years when that college had its best teams, my aunt attended a number of games (*on Saturday*) because, I assume, she wanted to be on hand when her little boy would be near-fatally injured. He was not more than five feet nine inches tall and probably weighed no more than 170 pounds. Leonard Carmichael, who was then chairman of the Department of Psychology at Brown, once got Oscar aside and expressed concern that he could be injured and was, perhaps, wasting his time playing football when he could start making a career in psychology, in which Professor Carmichael had concluded Oscar had shown considerable aptitude.

Oscar was directly important in my life. Toward the end of the first semester of my first year in junior high school, Oscar, home from college for a few days, visited our family. He interrogated my mother about the courses I was taking and was horrified to learn that I was enrolled in the commercial curriculum, taking such courses as typing, junior business training, etc. He told my mother that if I stayed in the commercial curriculum I would not be admitted to college. My mother was aghast and took action. A few weeks later, at the beginning of the next semester, I found myself taking Latin, ancient history, and algebra.

I do not have to relate more anecdotes to make the point that being Jewish was inextricably interwoven with attitudes toward intellectual accomplishment. To separate the one from the other was impossible. This did not mean that being Jewish meant that one was smart or capable of intellectual accomplishments, but it meant that one had respect for such strivings. Respect is too weak a word to convey the force and role of these attitudes. It is like saying that we have respect for breathing. We did not have to learn these attitudes in any consciously deliberate way. We had no choice in the matter, just as we had no choice in choosing our parents. As children, we did not have to verbalize these attitudes to ourselves, we would not have known how. The word *attitudes* is a poor one to describe what and how we absorbed what we did. We learned those attitudes in as "natural" a way as learning to like lox and bagels, gefilte fish, or knishes.

How do we account for the strength and frequency of these aspects of Jewishness? Please note that I am not asking how to account for individuals like myself or my mother and father or my cousins, but rather why these aspects are characteristics of Jews as a group. This is, initially, at least, a cultural, not a psychological, question. It is a question which directs us, among other things, to history and tradition and requires the adoption of a time perspective quite different from what we ordinarily use when our focus is on a single individual or generation. Obviously, if these aspects of Jewishness have been manifested for generations and centuries, the outlines of an answer to my question become clear—and I do not confuse clarity of outline with complexity of the substantive answer. These aspects, when looked upon in the context of the sweep of social-cultural history, have always characterized Jewish life. Indeed, when one looks at my question from this time perspective, one ends up by asking another question: So what else is new? Or, one becomes intrigued by individual Jews who do not possess these characteristics, whose mental breathing apparatus inexplicably did not take in ingredients ever present in his social-cultural atmosphere.

The aspects of Jewishness I have thus far discussed are not understandable by looking only at the present or near past. That is an obvious point which needed to be said in order to make a second one: *These aspects have been and will continue to be immune to change in any short period of time, by which I mean a minimum of a century.* Leaving aside Hitler's "final solution" as well as other types of world

64

catastrophes, I can think of no set of circumstances in which these aspects of Jewishness would disappear or be noticeably diluted in less than several or scores of generations. These circumstances could not be casual or indirect, they would have to be extremely potent and persistent. More of this later when I question the rationale behind the expectation that certain consequences of some aspects of blackishness can be changed noticeably in a decade or so, or that if blacks and whites differ on tests, one can ignore the relation of these differences to differences in the psychological core of blackishness and whiteishness, or that when you have equated a group of blacks and whites on an intelligence test or on a measure of academic achievement you have controlled for the most influential psychological determinants of intellectual performance in real life. (It's like saying that everybody is equal before the law, the person on welfare as well as the millionaire. There *is* a difference between facts and the truth.)

Now to another aspect of Jewishness to which I have alluded: the knowledge (it is not a feeling, it is phenomenologically a fact) that one is in a hostile world. This was crystal clear in my parents' and grandparents' generations. Their thinking went like this: Built into the mental core of every non-Jew is a dislike of and an enmity toward Jews. Yes, there were some nice Gentiles and up to a point you could trust and work with them, but let any conflict or dissension enter into the relationship and you would find that core of hatred asserting itself. It might not be verbalized, but, nonetheless, you could count on it. In the end, and there is always an end, you would get it in the neck—no ifs, ands, or buts. I have long felt that their resistance to mixed marriages—and the word *resistance* does not begin to convey the bitterness and strength of the feelings—was less a consequence of religion or clannishness than it was of the fear of physical injury to or destruction of one's child. To say they mistrusted the non-Jewish world is to reveal a genius for understatement. And if you tried to reason with them it was no contest because they could overwhelm you with history. They could marshall evidence from past centuries, as well as events in their own lives, with a rapidity, force, and cogency that doctoral students in history must fantasize about when they approach their orals. If you get a kick out of unproductive arguments I suggest you specialize in combating history with logic and goodwill— the kicks are endless. (If orthodox Jews are unavailable, try it with blacks, who have more kinship to Jews in this respect than they know.) If an aspect of you is poignantly and consciously rooted in history, you are not a candidate for attitude change. We would have had a more solid and realistic foundation for our efforts at social change if American social psychology had dealt with historically rooted, conscious attitudes of historically rooted groups. At the very least, it might have provided a more realistic time perspective about the attainment of the goals of these efforts.

What about me and my generation who, unlike our parents and grandparents, were born in this country with its traditions of opportunity and freedom? Did we possess the aspect of Jewishness that says this is a hostile world, even though "objectively" we grew up in a social environment radically different from that of previous generations? The very fact that our family had been created in this country and not in a European one meant that it would be different from what went before. You could write for years about the differences and when you were all through and began to list the similarities you would soon be listing the aspect "This is a hostile world for Jews." Some anecdotes from my adult life: When in 1938 I applied for admission to graduate school the knotty question was whether or not I would lie about being Jewish. Those were the days when you were asked for your religion and a photograph. They also wanted to know your father's occupation. So if I told them my father was a cutter of children's dresses, that I was Jewish, plus the fact that I would be graduated from an unrecognized college (Dana College, renamed the University of Newark, housed then in the former Feigenspan Brewery) what would be my chances? The point is not what was objectively true but the strength of my feeling that my application would be read by people hostile to Jews. The strength of my feeling and its automatic and indiscriminate application were not justified, but it is the hallmark of historically rooted attitudes of historically rooted groups that there is a discrepancy between external conditions and subjective impressions. (This is true for blacks in regard to whites, as it is for the Irish in regard to the English, etc.) The fact that these attitudes receive periodic reinforcement is sufficient to maintain their strength and indiscriminateness. For example, why does a colleague of mine still have in his possession a letter written to him in 1939 by a most eminent person who was then chairman of the department of psychology of a prestigious university? I have seen the letter. It is a remarkable but not surprising document because it says that although my colleague had all the paper credentials to be admitted to the doctoral program, he should think hard about coming because, as a Jew, he would not be able to be placed in a teaching job. A list of names is given of Jewish students who finished their doctorates in that department but who could not get jobs. Come, the letter says, but only if you regard it as an "intellectual adventure" and not as preparation for a career. How complicated a theory do we need to understand why my colleague, like myself, generalized our expectation of discrimination indiscriminately?

I lived in a radically different world than my parents and grandparents. I differed from them in countless important ways, but I differed not at all from them in the possession of this aspect of Jewishness. When I was finishing graduate school in 1942, there were two other students, and good friends (Jorma Niven, Harry Older), who were also going into the job market. To avoid competition among us, we did not apply for jobs at the same colleges or universities. Jorma and Harry were not Jewish, but they understood what was at stake when I wondered whether on my vita I should note that I was Jewish and so avoid interviews at places that did not look kindly on Jews. The point of these anecdotes is not to say something about the external world or even my perception of it but rather the pervasiveness and strength of my psychological radar about Jewishness, a constantly tuned instrument that was always at work and always sighting "objects" about which I had to decide whether they were friend or foe. But why do I say *was*? It is as true of me today as it was then, and with far less justification. My external world has changed dramatically within my lifetime, it has changed even more in relation to my parents' world, and yet that radar continues to work as if the external world has not changed.

A year ago when I was at a social gathering at Yale's Hillel, the Rabbi told me, in confidence and with that all too familiar mixture of pride and fear, that approximately one-third of all students at Yale were Jewish. He did not have to put into words (or even bother to look at me to see if I understood his message) that this information should not be bandied about because it might arouse the envy and enmity of non-Jews. You might expect such an attitude in a rabbi but not in me, but such an expectation simply ignores what fine-tuned, efficient processes and mechanisms cultural transmission consists of, insuring that the most central aspects of our sense of identity are independent of choice and changes in our external world.

I have known scores of Jews of my generation who have visited Israel. They were heterogeneous in many respects so that if you administered to them every psychological test that has ever been standardized, I predict you would find that, intelligence tests and political attitudes aside, the scores would be distributed in a fairly normal fashion. With no exception, every one of them spontaneously described the feeling—compounded of surprise, disbelief, relief, and security—they had in response to the fact that "everyone there is Jewish." As one of them said in deep puzzlement: "Even though I knew everyone was Jewish, I found that I continued to ask myself whether this or that person was Jewish. It was very unsettling at times." There are some attitudinal radars that cannot be turned off, because they have no off-on switch. These visitors shared another reaction, this one compounded of respect, envy, and pride and put by one of them in this way: "They have no fear. They don't care what the rest of the world thinks and does. They are prepared to fight and they have no doubt who will win in the end." To the non-Israeli Jew, "in the end" meant and still means getting it in the neck; to the Israeli it means quite the reverse. It took several generations of Israeli sabras, with an assist from Hitler, to effect a change in attitude. Put more correctly: It took all of that for a millenia-old identification to reassert itself. It was all right now to identify with David because one had to, and like David, but unlike those at Masada, the Goliath would be defeated. How strange this is to the American Jew. How strange it would be to the Israeli to learn about my reaction to an item in last week's *Yale Daily* that 50% of this year's Phi Beta Kappas were Jewish. He would have difficulty understanding my unreflective fear that this would not sit well in the minds of many non-Jews.

What about the younger generation of Jews in our society? Is this aspect of Jewishness in them or has it been eroded? As best as I can determine, this core of Jewishness is in them despite obvious changes in our society. When I asked a group of Jewish students about this, they looked at me as only smart-smart teen-agers can look at dumb-dumb professors, and one of them said: "In high school I read *The Wall*. There *was* the 1967 six-day war. And when I apply to medical school I know the chances of Jews have been decreased because they will take more minority people. How are we supposed to feel when we read that an African leader is sorry that Hitler did not win and that some black groups in our country seem to talk in the same way?" Toward the end of the discussion a young woman said, somewhat hostilely: "Because my parents were like you. What did *you* tell your daughter about going with or marrying a non-Jew?" A bull's-eye! Her comments recalled to me the time our family of three was about to leave our house to begin our first trip abroad. Just as we were ready to leave, my daughter (who then was 10) said she had forgotten something and went upstairs to get it. The "it" turned out to be a chain to which was attached a gold star of David. No, my wife and I had not given it to her because we are not religious.[1] It had been given to her by a Catholic nun who was head of an agency to which I had

---

[1] Jewishness, at least for many Jews in our society, is independent of religiousness, a fact which many rabbis keep complaining about, because they believe that when the two are experienced as independent, it will, over time, result in the disappearance of both. That they are experienced as independent was seen during the Israeli-Arab six-day war in 1967, as thousands of American Jews who had no interest in or commitment to Judaism spontaneously gave money for the support of Israel. The generosity of support is perhaps less relevant than the anxiety they felt about the threat to the continuation of Jewishness, not to the religion of their ancestors.

been a consultant, but that is another story, albeit a quite relevant one.

Before continuing, let me summarize what I have tried to say:

1. There are certain attitudinal characteristics which are part of the core of Jewishness. What is notable is their frequency and strength.

2. These characteristics are a kind of "second nature," learned, absorbed, and inculcated with all the force, subtleness, and efficiency of the processes of cultural transmission.

3. To understand the frequency and strength of these characteristics requires a time perspective of centuries.

4. Similarly, these characteristics could not be extinguished or diluted in strength except over very long periods of time. What centuries have produced will not quickly change even under external pressures.

5. It is impossible to understand and evaluate intellectual performance of groups without taking account of each group's attitudes toward such activity. This is an obvious point to anyone who has engaged in clinical work, and it has received substantial support in the research literature. It is no less valid a point when one deals with the intellectual performance of historically rooted groups and their historically rooted attitudes. (Women's liberation groups, now and in the distant past, understood this point quite well. The original title of this article was "Jewishness, Blackishness, Femaleness, and the Nature-Nurture Controversy.")

I have no difficulty accepting the notion that intelligence has its genetic components, nor do I have difficulty with the idea that different groups may possess different patterns of abilities. It would require mental derangement of a most serious sort to deny that different groups get different scores on various tests of intelligence. But I have the greatest difficulty understanding how anyone can come to a definitive conclusion in these matters based on studies which assume that what culture and history have created can be changed in a matter of years or decades. What combination of ignorance and presumption, what kind of understanding of human history does one have to possess to accept the hypothesis that the central psychological core of *historically* rooted groups can markedly change in a lifetime? It is a fact that Jews as a group score high on intelligence tests, do well on achievement tests, and are disproportionately represented in the professions and academia. It may be true that this is in part a consequence of selective survival and breeding over the centuries. But if one invokes the law of parsimony (not for the purposes of denying a hypothesis or preventing anyone from pursuing a particular line of research) for the purpose of assigning weights to variables on the basis of what we know about culture, one must conclude that the transmission of Jewishness from generation to generation has been fantastically successful —a view of "success" understood but probably not shared by those approaching their deaths in the Nazi holocaust, the Spanish Inquisition, and countless other Jew-murdering periods in history. My genes have a long history, an indisputable fact. My Jewishness also has a long history, another indisputable fact. At this point in time we know far more about my Jewishness than about my genes. When as a society we mount programs of social amelioration, I would prefer to act on the basis of the known, recognizing that I will not be alive to know the ultimate outcome.

BLACKISHNESS

What I have to say about "blackishness" has been foreshadowed by my description of certain aspects of Jewishness.[2] Jews and blacks share the characteristic "this is a hostile world." Some would argue that the sensitivity of blacks to anticipated hostility is stronger than it is in Jews. I am not sure this is the case, although some blacks and Jews would consider it self-evidently true. The more I talk to Jews about this, the more I am impressed by two things: how strong this aspect is and how much they want to believe that it isn't strong. Their self-report about its workings is discrepant with its strength. I stick with this point because it is instructive about what happens when two historically rooted attitudes contradict each other: "This is a hostile world" and "This is a society free of prejudice." In any event, this aspect of blackishness (in white society) is historically rooted and will be immune to change except over a long, long period of time. Blacks, of course, are absolutely correct when they say that an equally long period of time will be required for whites to overcome *their* historically rooted attitudes toward blacks.

In our society, at least, blackishness has not had at its core unbounded respect for book learning and the acquisition of academically soaked, cognitive skills. Just as when the Jews in Egypt were slaves, did manual labor, and could only hope for survival and dream of freedom, so in black culture, intellectuality or bookishness (call it

---

[2]Obviously, I cannot talk about blackishness with the affective nuance and depth of knowledge and experience that I can talk about Jewishness, nor is it necessary that I try or important that I cannot do justice to an equally complex cultural-psychological core. Sufficient for my purpose is that I pinpoint certain communalities and differences and their significance for the nature-nurture controversy.

what you will) has been far from the top on the priority list. As groups, Jews and blacks could not be more far apart than on the degree to which their cultures are suffused with "intellectuality." On intellegence tests Jews get higher scores than blacks.[3] *From my perspective, the important question is not how to explain the difference but why the difference is not greater.* This reminds me of Goddard's description of the Kallikak culture and his use of it as proof of Kallikak mental inferiority passed on from generation to generation. From his description of that encapsulated culture, one might conclude that the Kallikaks were a biologically superior group, that is, anyone who could grow up and survive in that culture must have been extremely well endowed constitutionally.

Over the past century, more and more blacks have "made it" in the intellectual arena, but they have represented a very small percentage of all blacks. It is my impression that compared even to three decades ago, more black children experience something akin to what I described of my childhood, but there is no basis at all for concluding that this has become a characteristic experience. What warrant is there in psychological theory and research that would lead to the expectation that the attitudinal core of blackishness could, under the most favorable conditions, be changed in less than scores of generations. And is there a psychologist who would argue that we have even remotely approximated "the most favorable conditions."

For me, the central question is how theories determine time perspective, that is, how one's conception of what man and society are determines one's time perspective about changing either? I have discussed this in connection with the problem of changing schools and creating new settings (Sarason, 1971, 1972). Two examples of what

---

[3]There was a time (decades ago) when Jews, like blacks today, were viewed as being mentally inferior because of inferior genetic endowment. I am indebted to my colleague, Edward Zigler (personal communication, 1973) for pointing out to me the anti-Jewish attitudes of the early eugenicists, particularly Galton and Pearson. In a manuscript he is preparing, Zigler states:

Pearson continually employed genetic arguments in his efforts to stem the immigration of Polish and Russian Jews into England, arguing that they were genetically inferior to the earlier settlers of the English nation. He concluded "Taken on the average, and regarding both sexes, this alien Jewish population is somewhat inferior physically and mentally to the native population. . . .

The anti-Jewish attitude of the early eugenicists finally culminated in the complete bastardization of the eugenics movement in Nazi Germany, where the "final solution" of dealing with "races" of inferior genetic stock was to murder them in gas ovens. It is interesting to note that less than 50 years after Pearson's assertion of the genetic inferiority of the Jews, another distinguished Englishman, C. P. Snow, argued that in light of the large number of Jewish Nobel laureates, the Jews must be a superior people. We thus see how tenuous indeed are those assertions that a particular group is inferior or superior.

I mean: What if someone came to us and asked why we cannot teach children to read in 24 hours? Assuming that we knew the person to be sane and we could control the tendency to throw him out of our office, what would we say? It would probably take us 24 hours of uninterrupted talk to explain how children develop physically, mentally, and socially; the inevitable social and interpersonal context in which learning takes place; the complexity of motivation and its vicissitudes; the knowledge and cognitive skills that are necessary for the productive assimilation and use of symbols; and the problems that can be created when external pressures do not take developmental stages readiness into account. Besides, we might ask this irritating ignoramus, Do you mean why can't we teach *a* child to read in 24 hours or do you mean a *group* of children in a classroom?

A second example: What if we went to a psychoanalyst friend and asked him really to level with us and explain how he justifies seeing *a* patient for one hour a day, four or five days a week, perhaps for two, three, four, or more years. Why does it take that long? Do you really believe, we ask him, that it takes that long to be helpful to someone? Aren't there quicker ways of giving help? Friend (?), he replies, there is much you do not understand. He then proceeds to summarize for us what the human organism is at birth, how its cognitive and affective equipment is organized and develops, the ways in which it becomes increasingly psychologically and physically differentiated, how it develops and utilizes a variety of coping mechanisms, the sources of inevitable internal and external conflict, the nature and strength of resistances to change, the relationship of all of this to the interpersonal dynamics of the nuclear family, and on and on depending on whether our psychoanalyst friend is summarizing Freud's *Introductory Lectures* or multivolumed collected works. (If he happens to be a true believer, we would also hear about patricide and the primal horde in the dawning history of mankind.) Now, he would say, you can begin to understand why psychoanalytic treatment takes so long. It is not that we desire to prolong it, but rather that our understanding of man requires it if we are to be able meaningfully to help somebody radically change accustomed ways of thinking and acting. Of course, he would admit, you can help troubled people in a shorter period of time by focusing only on the elimination of symptoms, but that is not our goal, which is to illuminate for our patients their psychological core and its dynamics, and we are not always successful.

I do not have to labor the point that one's conception of a problem or process determines one's time perspective about how to influence or change it. The relationship may be grossly invalid either because one's conception is faulty, or one's time perspective poorly deduced, or both, but the fact remains that there is always a relationship. In my opinion, the failure or inability to confront this relationship in a systematic and realistic way is one of the most frequent sources of personal disillusionment and conflict, as it is also one of the central defects in most social science theorizing. Is it not amazing how many social scientists reacted to the Supreme Court desegregation decision in 1954 as if it really meant that desegregation was ended, or would be ended in a matter of a decade or so? Is it not equally amazing how many people really believed that if disadvantaged groups, like the blacks, were provided new and enriched educational experiences they would as a group blossom quickly in terms of conventional educational and intellectual criteria? Is it not pathetic how eager we were to believe that we possessed the knowledge to justify these expectations? What combination of ignorance and arrogance permitted people to proclaim that if we delivered the right kinds of programs and spent the appropriate sums of money we could quickly undo what centuries had built up? When the expectations that powered these efforts were obviously not being fulfilled, what permitted some people to conclude that perhaps the victim was in some ways different from (less endowed than) those in the dominant society? Why were they so ready to "blame the victim" instead of the thinking from which derived such an unrealistic time perspective? And again I must ask: What is there in man's history and in the corpus of social science knowledge which contradicts the statement that few things are as immune to quick changes as the historically rooted, psychological core of ethnic and racial groups? Jewishness and blackishness are products, among other things (and I assume there *are* other things), of social and cultural history, and their psychological cores will successfully resist short-term efforts aimed at changing them.

In one of his syndicated columns, William F. Buckley, Jr. (*New Haven Journal Courier*, March 20, 1969) has provided support of my thesis: needless to say, he does this unknowingly. Buckley quoted approvingly from an article by Ernest van den Haag:

> The heart of Mr. van den Haag's analysis, so critically useful at the present moment, should be committed to memory before the ideologists of racism take the Jensen findings and mount a campaign of I-told-you-soism with truly ugly implications. Van den Haag asked himself:
>
> Q. Suppose the average native intelligence of Negroes is inferior to that of whites. Would that mean that Negroes are inferior to whites?
>
> A. One may regard others as inferior to oneself, or to one's group, on the basis of any criterion, such as mating, eating, drinking or language habits, religious practices, or competence in sports, business, politics, art

or finally, by preferring one's own type, quality or degree of intelligence, skin or hair color and so forth.

By selecting appropriate criteria each group can establish the inferiority of others, and its own superiority. . . . The selection of criteria for superiority or inferiority is arbitrary, of course . . . I do not believe that intelligence is any more relevant to judgments of inferiority than, say, skin color is.

If Negroes on the average turn out to have a genetically lower learning ability than whites in some respects, e.g. the manipulation of abstract symbols, and if one chooses this ability as the ranking criterion, it would make Negroes on the average inferior to some whites and superior to others. Suppose four-fifths of Negroes fall into the lower half of intelligence distribution. Chances are that, say, one-third of the whites will too. Hence, if intelligence is the criterion, the four-fifths of the Negro group would be no more "inferior" than the one-third of the white group. Judgments of inferiority among whites are rarely based solely on intelligence. There certainly are many people who do not rank high on intelligence tests but are, nonetheless, preferable, and preferred, to others who do. I know of no one who selects his associates—let alone friends—purely in terms of intelligence. God knows, we certainly do not elect to political office those who are most intelligent. I would conclude that whatever we may find out about Negro intelligence would not entail any judgment about general inferiority.

Buckley concluded the column with these words aimed at those who "by their dogmatic insistence on 'equality' at every level succeeded in persuading typical Americans to put far too great an emphasis on 'intelligence'":

Add to these observations the Christian point: namely that all men are equal in the truest sense of the word, and the findings of Dr. Jensen are placed in perspective. But it will take time to undo the damage brought by the ideologization of science during the reign of American liberalism.

It will take time to undo the damage! Mr. Buckley seems to have grasped the principle that historically rooted attitudes do not change quickly with time or evidence. He knows this to be true for political attitudes, that is, the liberal or conservative ideology. He knows this to be true of himself as a historically minded Catholic. If he cannot apply the principle to the nature and consequences of blackishness in our society, we should not be harsh, because it is a principle that unless rooted firmly in self-knowledge *as well as* knowledge of the force and processes of cultural transmission cannot be applied as a general principle.

Mr. Buckley's column was his answer to a study sponsored by the Anti-Defamation League of the B'nai Brith. It is understandable that he paid attention to the study and not to its sponsor. If he had asked why this Jewish group sponsored such a study, he would have gotten the conventional response: For obvious historical reasons, Jews are not indifferent to any form of religious, racial, or ethnic discrimination; if they do not defend *any* victim of discrimination, their own vulnerability to discrimination is increased; discrimination is a wound-producing act, the effects of which never heal in the lifetime of the victim. Mr. Buckley knows all this and knows it well. But what Mr. Buckley does not know, and what many Jews sense but would have difficulty conceptualizing and articulating, is that historically rooted discrimination (its causes and consequences) is immune to change by efforts based on our accustomed short-time perspective. I suspect that the guilt of whites in relation to blacks has to do with the intuitive feeling that black freedom is a long, long way off. I also suspect that the anger of blacks toward whites has the same source. The future is determining the present.

Why say all of this? The answer, which goes back 30 years to when I started work at the Southbury Training School, is suggested in two statements. First, if a neighbor's child had an IQ of 180 and strangled a dog to death, we would not say he did it *because* he had an IQ of 180. Second, if that neighbor's child had an IQ of 60, our prepotent response, our *act of discrimination*, would be to point to the IQ of 60 as the etiological agent without which the strangling would not have taken place.[4] This pernicious double-standard way of thinking, the essence of discrimination, is so ingrained in us that when we recognize our logical error we feel helpless about how we should proceed to think and act. Life is so much easier when we, the experts, like most other people, can "blame the victim" for what he is and "is" means that he has a low IQ, and what more do we need to know to understand him? Why complicate our thinking by confronting

---

[4]We blame "bad" things on a low IQ, and we explain "good" ones by a high IQ, differences in language which are the hallmark of cultural influence. It is such a part of our thinking, it all appears so self-evident, that we cannot recognize the diverse ways in which these cultural influences work, for example, their self-fulfilling tendencies. For example, 25 years ago, Catherine Cox Miles, a long-time colleague of Lewis Terman, told me that nowhere in his write-up of his studies of "gifted" California boys and girls did Terman indicate the amount of time he spent helping his subjects get into college and graduate school, and obtain jobs. There was absolutely no chicanery involved. It was so self-evident to him that a high IQ was the cause of superior accomplishment that he could not recognize that he was an intervening variable, that is, that he, Lewis Terman, was a reflection and guardian of certain cultural values.

the fact that the act of constructing and using tests is both a reflection and a determinant of cultural attitudes and deeply rooted ways of thinking which, as long as they go unrecognized, guarantee that facts will be confused with truth? Why get into these messy issues when you can talk about genetics? Of course, we should study the genetics of intelligence (high, low, black, white) but, unless I misread the history of genetics, productive theorizing about genotypes follows upon clearly described, stable phenotypes. In regard to the genetics of intelligence, we are far from the point at which we can say that we have a well-described, stable phenotype. The one thing we can say with assurance is that our concepts of intelligence are value laden, culture and time bound, and deficient in cross-cultural validity. *It has not even been demonstrated that the level of problem-solving behavior in nontest situations is highly correlated with the level of similar types of problem-solving processes in the standardized test situations* (Sarason & Doris, 1969). And, as I have tried to demonstrate in this article, relatively little attention has been paid either to the different ways in which attitudes toward intellectual activity are absorbed by and inculcated in us, or to how the presence or absence of these group attitudes has behind it the force of decades or centuries.

I began with a story about my father and I shall end with one. He was in the hospital recovering from an operation. I visited him on one day, and my brother visited him on the next. The nurse asked my father what work his sons did. When he told her that they were both professors of psychology, she semifacetiously asked him: "Mr. Sarason, how come *you* have two sons like that?" My sister reported that my father, without a moment's hesitation and with the most profound seriousness, replied: "Don't you know that smartness sometimes skips generations?" The nature and force of the processes of cultural transmission never skip generations, particularly when their ways have been finely honed over the centuries. They will not be quickly blunted. I excuse my father for not knowing this (although he may have known it). I cannot excuse this in the participants of the recent nature-nurture controversy. There is a point when one must regard the consequences of ignorance as sinful, and that point was reached for the advocates of nurture when they expected that the core of blackishness would quickly change; and it was reached by the advocates of nature when they concluded that the overall failure of compensatory programs demonstrated the significance of genetic factors on which new programs should be based. With friends like that, the blacks need not waste time worrying about enemies, a lesson Jews learned well over the centuries.

REFERENCES

Sarason, S. B. *The culture of the school and the problem of change.* Boston: Allyn & Bacon, 1971.
Sarason, S. B. *The creation of settings and the future societies.* San Francisco: Jossey-Bass, 1972.
Sarason, S. B., & Doris, J. *Psychological problems in mental deficiency.* (4th ed.) New York: Harper & Row, 1969.

Commentary to
Chapters 7 and 8

Earlier I explained why this volume does not contain any article from the Test Anxiety Project, how that project delayed my moving in new directions, and how terminating that project radically altered my view of myself and psychology. One of the things I learned about myself was that my strong need to feel creative would not (should not) permit me to stick with a problem beyond a few years. It was not that I had to move on after milking the problem dry but rather that, once I felt that I had grasped, formulated, and discussed the problem—once I felt that I had correctly come to the core of the problem—the process of empirical follow-through held little interest for me. One such problem was the way in which highly educated people—the professionals—experienced the relationship between work and aging. That problem came to occupy me shortly before I gave up the directorship of the Yale Psycho-Educational Clinic. It was a deeply personal problem in two respects. My parents, both non-professionals, were aging and sick, and caring for them was a mammoth task that opened my eyes to certain features of our society. I was aging and increasingly had to face my own way of pushing my mortality further into the future. To feel creative is to feel rejuvenated, to feel young, to feel that the end is far off in the future.

Initially, it was my intention to study old people and our society, but for a variety of reasons I did not see that that focus would not be satisfying to me, partly because I was so occupied with the relationships in my own life between the sense of aging (the sense of time passing) and the nature of work. I floundered for a couple of years until I realized that, over the next few decades, our society would have more highly educated old people than any society past or present. How would these people experience aging? How would their expectations about satisfaction from work be fulfilled or frustrated in our society? Once I started to ask these kinds of questions, I came to see the dilemmas of the "one life–one career imperative." Our society had made it much easier to change marriage partners than to change careers. It all started to come together and was formulated in the article that follows. That was prologue to the book Work, Aging, and Social Change: Professionals and the One Life–One

Career Imperative *(1977, 1). Because it illustrates in a very personal way the theme of the book, the article is followed by a chapter from the book, "Career Change: An Autobiographical Fragment."*

7

Aging and the Nature of Work

In Western society, at least, the view that the nature of work poses serious personal and social problems is not new. The age of the machine, nurtured by the science, technology, and invention ushered in by the Renaissance and growing rapidly as a result of the industrial revolution, was early on seen as a mixed blessing. One part of the blessing was wrapped up in the concept of progress: man's capacity through reason (impersonal, objective, and implacable) to understand and use the laws of nature so as to lead, slowly but surely, to an earthly heaven. The other part was in the nature of a curse: the means whereby this earthly heaven was to be achieved would come to dominate man, alienating him from himself (his "true" nature) and others (the "natural" order of social living). Whatever criticisms can be directed at Marx's heroic intellectual effort to conceptualize the past in order to factor out the harbingers of an inevitable future, no one has seriously contested his analysis of how the age of the machine has adversely transformed the nature of work and, therefore, man's consciousness. Just as in the 1954 desegregation decision when the Supreme Court contended that segregation had adverse effects both on the segregatee and the segregator, almost a century earlier Marx was making the identical point about capitalists and workers. It is beyond the scope of this article to examine the history of the changing nature of work. The interested reader should consult the writings of Lewis Mumford, and also Thomas Green's (1968) illuminating *Work, Leisure, and the American Schools*. We allude to history not only as a caution against the parochialism that is a consequence of the ahistorical stance but, as we hope to make clear shortly, because history

S. B. Sarason, E. K. Sarason, and P. Cowden, "Aging and the Nature of Work," *American Psychologist* 30, no. 5 (May 1975): 584–592. Copyright 1975 by the American Psychological Association. Reprinted by permission.

ill prepared us to recognize that work has become a problem for many *professionals* who heretofore were viewed as the chosen few exempt from feelings of boredom, lack of challenge, and sense of worth. Professionals have long sold themselves and others the view that it was the factory worker who was victimized by the nature of his work.[1] In Green's terms, the man in the factory *labored*; the professional *worked*. And the difference between laboring and working (in Green's terms) is no different than that between Marx's industrial slave and capitalist exploiter. One was stamped or branded *by* his work; the other put his stamp or brand *on* his work.

A brief comment is in order about the title of this article, if only to note and explain why we will have relatively little to say about aging. A basic hypothesis in our approach is that one's relationship to work is one of the important determinants of how present and future time is experienced, that is, one's sense of the passage of time. This sense of the passage of time inevitably shapes and becomes one's psychological sense of aging. It follows that there should be no significant correlation between the psychological sense of aging and biological processes, although at some point they become intertwined. When we use such words as *aging* or the *aged*, we usually implicitly assume that the awareness of aging begins at or after mid-life. When we see in ourselves or others the visible signs of biological aging, it takes no particular psychological wisdom to assume that they have psychological correlates. In our culture, at least, we do not think of people as aging or aged until we literally see the visible signs of biological aging. We are not accustomed to thinking of the psychological sense of aging in developmental terms, as an internal set of attitudes shaped by experiences of various kinds in a culture suffused with reminders of the passage of time—reminders that almost always are wittingly or unwittingly calculated to make us view that passage in dysphoric terms. But once it becomes obvious that the psychological sense of aging has its developmental roots in our experience of the passage of time—once we unlearn the habit of thinking in terms of a

---

[1] There is a serious problem in interpreting findings about job satisfaction from available studies, especially because almost all of the studies are based on questionnaire data. To express dissatisfaction or boredom with, or a waning interest in, one's work—*particularly if one's work is judged by society as fascinating and important as in the case of many professions* —is no easy matter. To face up to such dissatisfaction is literally to question what one *is* and to have to justify continuing as one has. It is no less difficult, upsetting, and propelling than to come to the realization that one no longer wishes to live with one's spouse. Our experience suggests that to talk candidly about one's relationship to one's work is as difficult as talking about one's sex life. We define ourselves, and are defined by others, by what we do: our work. To question this definition produces internal conflict, in part precisely because we know that we have come to see ourselves quite differently than others do.

high correlation between the psychological sense of aging and chrono-
logical age—we can direct our attention to those things that influence
the content and vicissitudes of the experience of the passage of time
and, therefore, the emerging sense of aging. And one of these important factors is one's experiences in the world of work: how one plans
for, enters, and experiences work. This is one factor, but it is very
complicated, related as it is to the major dimensions by which our
society is organized, for example, economic, class, sex, education,
the family unit, religion, race, etc. In this article, therefore, we restrict ourselves to some of the considerations directing our exploratory
studies.

POLICY AND POPULATIONS

When this project began to be developed in 1972, our sole focus was
on the problems of older people. As we read the literature, talked
with numerous professionals, and drew upon a variety of personal experiences, several things became apparent or started to emerge. The
literature was overwhelmingly clinical and, not surprisingly, so were
and are the myriads of public programs to which it gave rise. Stated
most simply: Old people had a lot of serious personal, social, financial,
housing, and medical problems, and society had an obligation to
alleviate their plight. There was, of course, a secondary preventive
thrust to these programs in that they aimed to avoid having existing
problems worsen and create new problems. It is fair to say that a
primary preventive approach was conspicuous by its absence, although
on the level of rhetoric it was given lip service. A second factor, related to the first, was the enormous and morally upsetting discrepancy
between defined needs and available resources, a characteristic en-
demic to the clinical endeavor. Frankly, as we became more involved
with aged individuals and their families, with settings we euphemis-
tically call *convalescent* or *nursing homes*, as well as with a medical
profession whose knowledge of attitudes toward the elderly quintessentially illustrate the pernicious aspects of the self-fulfilling prophecy,
we had inordinate difficulty maintaining our own stability. For the
first year we found ourselves deeply focused on examination of
policies and programs (retirement, age discrimination, housing, trans-
portation, public education): their underlying assumptions, the
cultural attitudes which powered them, implementation, and
effectiveness.
    Our disquietude had another source: our bias in favor of a
preventive-developmental approach to human problems. We were

aware that, despite our bias, we were being drawn more and more into a remedial framework which, given our project resources, seemed inefficient if not ludicrous. It should go without saying that anyone whose efforts are directed to clinical work—be it with the elderly, children, or any other group in need—does not have to justify his activities (their effectiveness is another issue). When you are in need and seek help, you are (or should be) grateful that clinicians exist. But when these needs are staggering in their frequency, and in varying ways and degrees reflect characteristics of our society, the limitations of an exclusively clinical approach are obvious (Sarason, 1974). This is especially true when the nature of and the rationale for the clinical approach hardly reflects a sensitivity to the larger social context.

It was both our bias and disquietude that opened our eyes and ears to "messages" to which we had been responding in terms as far removed from aging as one could imagine. Embedded as we were in a university, interacting constantly with students of widely differing backgrounds and interests, trying hard to comprehend their articulated dissatisfactions with society's past, present, and future, puzzled by their bleak projections of themselves over their life span, fascinated by the different lifestyles they were trying—at some point we attached several significances to these observations that gave expression to our bias and allowed us to think differently about aging.

A sizable fraction of students feared being *trapped* in life. This was phrased and fantasied in different ways by students, but there was the common theme that their postcollege future would be a downhill experience. This did not mean (for most, at least) that they did not wish it would be otherwise or that they would not strive to make it otherwise, but rather that they feared the probabilities were high that they would become mired in an "establishment" existence tantamount to a slow death. They spoke about the future with a depressive and oppressive anxiety similar to that which one hears in the elderly. What we are trying to say is captured in the title of a book written by an undergraduate, *Growing Up Old In The Sixties* (Maynard, 1973). When we would ask students to write about "How young or old do you feel?" a surprising number said that they did not feel young but, rather (surprising *to them*), old. When we would interrogate them, sometimes in long no-holds-barred discussion, about how they would account for such a feeling—why they viewed the future so bleakly—they were not very articulate until they forced us (the interrogators) to face the fact that we grew up in very different times; that is, we grew up when it was possible to believe that society could be significantly reformed, whereas they were growing up when such a possibility was virtually nonexistent.

In light of the above, it was not surprising that so many students thought about and planned for a career with reluctance, anxiety, and even anger. As one student put it: "Why blame us for trying to postpone dying?" Or as another student put it: "Why should it be puzzling to you that we have serious doubts about striving for something that may kill us?" We make no claims about the generality of these feelings and attitudes except to say that we obtained them from undergraduate and graduate students in different universities. Obviously, there are many students who do not share these feelings and attitudes. Although it is important, it is not crucial for our purposes here to estimate the percentage of students who do have these reactions. Of the countless colleagues, at Yale and elsewhere, with whom we have discussed these matters, not one doubted that these attitudes were frequent. And, let us not overlook another obvious fact: the number of students who have dropped out of school and society not available to us for questioning.

When we put our experiences with college students together with our knowledge of public policy and programming for the elderly, we were struck by something we consider of enormous significance. *Theory and practice in regard to the elderly are almost totally determined by the perceived characteristics of those who are now elderly. In three or more decades we will have the most formally educated aged population any society has ever had. There is good reason to believe that becoming aged will pose for them and society problems radically different and potentially more personally and socially disruptive than is the case with today's elderly population.*[2] Once the "obvious" dawned on us it reinforced our determination to pursue a developmental course of investigation. It also gave substantive direction to the kinds of studies we had to undertake. These studies are in their initial phases. Their thrust is best communicated by the considerations underlying them.

CONSIDERATIONS

Our studies, for a while at least, will concentrate on people who have had or are now obtaining a higher education. This focus, as we have suggested, is dictated not only by the relative narrowness in the literature on work but also by the knowledge that over the next few

---

[2] In April 1974, after this article was prepared, the Federal Administration on Aging circulated guidelines and priorities for support of model projects of national scope. There is no doubt from these documents that policy and programs are being viewed only in terms of those who are currently elderly. One should be thankful, of course, for this concern, but in terms of national programs and policies it is amazingly shortsighted.

decades an increasing segment of our society will have had some degree of college experience.

1. *The process of making a career choice is the first significant confrontation with the sense of aging, involving as it does the knowledge or belief that such a decision is fateful because it determines how the rest of one's life will be "filled in."* It is a "moment of truth" kind of problem which makes for varying degrees of vacillation, postponement, and anxiety because the choice involves numerous factors: strength of interests, familial relationships and pressures, economic factors (personal and national), love and peer relationships, time perspective, and how one reads and structures the future. The need for independence and autonomy comes face-to-face with societal pressure to conform, not the least of which is that one feels one *has* to make a decision at a particular point in time. One can no longer sample from the smorgasbord of opportunity; one *must* choose and live with the choice. There are, of course, individuals, probably small in number, who long have known what they were going to do; they are viewed by some with envy, by others with derision, and by still others with an effete attitude that seems to be saying "anyone who willingly and joyously enters this real world with the expectation of happiness has postponed his moment of truth." However one conceptualizes the process of career choice, one cannot ignore that at this particular time in our society the process is for many suffused with dysphoric anticipations about what may be symbolically called *dying*. It is not only a matter of "am I making the right or wrong choice" but, for many, "will society allow me to be the kind of person I want to be, regardless of choice?" The locus of control is perceived as external rather than internal. This has probably been the case for past decades, but it was accompanied by the belief that by striving, diligence, and maneuvering one could lick the odds. This accompaniment is much less in evidence today.

2. Since World War II, and in no small measure because of it, the number of new fields and career possibilities has escalated. Just as during this same period it has become possible to easily travel and vacation any place on this earth, a young person today is aware of a much greater array of career possibilities than was true in his parents' generation. *Both within and among fields the choices are many. Students are aware of this as they are of the stubborn fact that they must make a choice. They are also aware that at the same time that society tells them that there are numerous directions available to them, the educational system (beginning in high school) is organized increasingly to pressure the student to narrow his choices.* In college they must choose *a* major, and in graduate and professional school they are also

forced to declare their choice. For example, a student does not apply to graduate school because he is interested in the field of psychology but rather because he has been required, formally or informally, to declare his special interest, e.g., clinical, physiological, social, personality, child, cognitive, industrial, educational, learning. Theoretically the options are many; in practice they are few. The discrepancy, for some students, arouses a strange mixture of sense of loss, the need to justify choice by eliminating dissonance, and a passive acceptance of fate's workings. For others the discrepancy is far less of a problem. By the time a student of either type has been in graduate or professional school for a year or more he already knows how narrow his horizons have become. This is especially true for that ever-increasing number of students who choose medicine or law because each of these fields was perceived as containing many more career options than other fields.

3. *For many reasons, chiefly demographic and economic, our society will increasingly contain individuals who will go through life knowing that they never were able to enter the career of their first choice.* There has always been a discrepancy between the number of graduate and professional school applications and openings. In recent years this discrepancy has become nothing short of scandalous. Not having the opportunity to enter the career of first choice need not be a tragedy, and undoubtedly there are some individuals who enter other careers that give them satisfactions. But for many the disappointment will be a festering irritant interacting with later frustrations to cloud present and future with the deprivations of the past. To go through life knowing that one's work is one's second or third choice must affect one's sense of the passage of time, how one justifies existence and looks to an ever-shortening future. The sense of worth has diverse sources, but few are as potent as how one regards one's work. It could be argued that the market place of life finds ways of compensating for disappointments; that is, an unsatisfied demand will be made up for by some substitute supply of compensation. But markets, economic and psychological, break down, sometimes with convulsive consequences. When we consider that our society will have an increasing number of educated people as well as an increasing number who will not have been "allowed" to pursue a primary interest, it is difficult to adopt an indifferent or positive stance. Rising expectations together with rising frustrations have a revolutionary potential which, when and if it becomes manifest, can take a retrograde rather than a progressive form.

4. *There has been an increase in the number of people who seek a career change, be that change within or between fields of work.*

There are no data on the frequency of such changes, but our observations, interviews, and some exploratory studies lead us to the conclusion that it is far from an infrequent phenomenon. The dynamics powering such changes are complicated and varied. The sought-for change can take place at any time after one has begun a career. Indeed, it is our impression that whereas it used to be a "midcareer crisis," it now can occur much earlier. Several factors have contributed to both the increased frequency and earlier timing of career changes. One of these factors is the emphasis placed on the social worth of one's work. It has always been the case that professionals were expected to experience their work as personally satisfying, its social worthiness being taken for granted. It is precisely the social worth of much professional work that has been called into question in recent years. The atomic bombing of Hiroshima, the generalized consequences of the turbulent sixties, the turmoil surrounding the Vietnam war—this train of events instigated in many professionals profound questioning about the significance of their work. If the questioning was not strong enough to produce wholesale career changes, it nevertheless placed the significance of work high on the social agenda. When individuals no longer believe in the inevitability of progress, when they see themselves and their work as perhaps contributing to the moral confusion, it is small wonder that some will seek to make radical changes in their work and life style. Another factor, no less important than the first, is that recent generations have expected more from their work, that is, that their work will and should always be challenging and novelty producing. That is to say, work should be intrinsically stimulating and productive of "self-actualization" or "personal growth." And can anyone doubt that the past few decades have seen a fantastic rise in the number of people who spend their time helping others to "grow," to recognize their "true selves," to be unafraid of change and novelty, and "to do their thing"? Ours is a time of conflicting and even contradictory tendencies: a new form of rugged individualism and a heightened sense of social responsibility. It was inevitable that these tendencies would have repercussions in the world of work in the form of an increase in career changes. The dynamics and their consequences are similar to those with respect to marriage and divorce. On the level of rhetoric, at least, it used to be that when one got married it was supposed to be forever, a view of the future supported by religion and law. And if one did not believe that marriages were made in heaven, there was no doubt that they could not easily be undone on earth. One was expected to make the best of the marriage. One life, one marriage partner. That, of course, has changed as it is changing in the world of work. It is true that our society has made it far easier to change marriage partners than to change careers, but that difference may well be in the process of being eroded. What is involved here is not only a changing set of attitudes toward work but to the experience of the passage of time in which dying and "imprisonment" are symbolically or literally somewhere in the background. To see one's self as remaining "unfulfilled" or "bored" or "locked in" in what is perceived as a world of endless possibilities in a finite, shortening life raises the conflict between activity and passivity to a very heightened level, higher, we think, than it has ever been before in our society.

Each of the above four statements could be elaborated into a book and, in fact, each has received extended comment and analysis from different perspectives in hundreds of books written in the past two decades. Despite these different perspectives there is agreement on one thing: Although their sources and dynamics have roots in the distant past and there have been and probably will be a waxing and waning in their surface manifestations, there has been a significant alteration in people's attitudes and values in regard to self, work, and social living. To some this alteration is prologue to social decay; to others it is prodromal to a better world in the making; to still others it is only confusion compounded of mystery and meaninglessness leading nowhere in particular. Without question, it is the younger generations who tend to pessimism, cynicism, and even nihilism. Their view of themselves in the future bears some startling similarities to what one frequently finds among the aged. Whereas many of the aged (or not so aged) look back and ask: *"Was* it worth it?" many younger people look forward and ask: *"Will* it be worth it?" And although these two questions have a complex of referents, the experience of work is among the most important.

The four statements have given and will give direction to a variety of initial studies on the process and phenomenology of career choice among college students: changes in attitudes toward the career and the future that take place in the course of graduate and professional education, the timing and frequency of career changes, and the ever developing awareness of the sense of the passage of time and its merging into the sense of aging. We do not doubt that our studies will cause us to change our conceptions in certain respects. Our initial data, however, confirm what we suspected in two very important respects. First, the years devoted to professional education are experienced as an ever-narrowing of horizons and options in which personal choice and style are compromised by the need to conform to externally set criteria of "success." For example, when one interviews students headed for law, medical, or graduate school, they have two major expectations: Either they see themselves as having boundless opportunities to absorb new knowledge and experience which will subsequently open all sorts of career possibilities to them in the near and distant future, or they recognize that there will or may be a conflict between what they hope and what they will be required to do, but somehow their internal compass for maintaining integrity will protect them (a subsegment of this group are those who truly view professional education with foreboding and no compass). When one interviews students near the end of their professional training, one is struck by their feeling that they have been "molded," have been forced to become "realistic," and that the options they once expected to be available to them have been reduced drastically. There is in many of them a quiet desperation, a knowledge that the status, capabilities, and satisfactions that society projects onto them, far from being balm, create in them a guilty unease. And when we find, as we have, that at least 20% of a sample of physicians explicitly express dissatisfaction with their careers, the forebodings of our younger interviewees cannot be viewed as without some merit.[3]

The second way in which our exploratory studies support what we and others have intuited is that the number of people who seek a career change is not small. Based on an analysis of graduate school applicants, and depending on how one defines career change, we found between 10% and 20% who were 25 years or older and sought a change. We have also become aware (by reading the advertising section for professional personnel in the *New York Times*) that within the past few years agencies have come into existence with the exclusive purpose of counselling professional individuals seeking a career change. We interviewed the director of one agency who told us that he could not keep up with requests for service, and his fee was not small. He was also in the process of setting up satellite offices in several other big cities. What the figures would be nationally or by the different professions we cannot say. We have been discussing individuals who are actively seeking a career change. We have no good basis for hazarding a guess as to how many people would like to change careers but take no active step to do so. In any event, we can no longer afford to reinforce the view that work dissatisfaction is peculiar to blue or

---

[3] These data were obtained by Victor Lieberman in a study not designed to get at job satisfaction, but three questions relevant to job satisfaction were added. These data are not reported in his write-up (Lieberman, 1974). The interviews were of necessity brief and there was a marked age discrepancy between the interviewer and the physicians. It was surprising, therefore, that 20% unambiguously expressed dissatisfaction with their work. Informal interviews with physicans we knew well—enabling us to ask direct and unambiguous questions —lead us to believe that 20% is an underestimate.

white collar workers. Terkel's (1974) book *Working* deservedly received a good deal of acclaim, but we fear that one of its unintended consequences will be to reinforce the belief that work is a major problem only for certain segments of the population.

Our discussions with diverse professionals have brought out a consideration deserving of special comment. It is what might be called the "How many times do you climb Mt. Everest?" phenomenon. Most simply put, it is the experience that one has successfully mastered one's "trade" but that is not sufficient reason to continue doing the same thing, albeit successfully, for the rest of one's life. It is not that the work is not intrinsically interesting but that it has lost some if not most of its novelty or challenging features. They enjoy the status and financial rewards that success has brought them but there is the nagging thought that there are other things they would like to try to be; and if, as they thought quite likely, they would not make a change (because in each instance of great loss in income) they may find their remaining years somewhat disappointing or empty. As has been pointed out elsewhere (Sarason, 1972), in the context of the nature of leadership, the consequences of success *because* one has mastered the job can have untoward consequences. There is a prepotent tendency to view job dissatisfaction as in part reflecting intrinsically negative features of the work *qua* work. But as a surgeon said to us: "Surgery *is* interesting. For a period of years it did fascinate me. I *am* a good surgeon. In fact, I'm a damned good one. So I'm good, so what? What I really want to do is to get into the history of medicine." This individual was in his middle years, but he, like others with whom we have talked, was voicing something similar to what younger interviewees were saying; that is, they did not want to feel that they were going to do one thing in life, to be walled in by narrow specialization.

Thus far in this article we have emphasized several major points, but chief among them has been that work is a problem for many highly educated, professional people and that many of today's would-be professionals view the world of work with critical questioning, doubts, and negative affect. The significance of these points, it should be remembered, lies in the indisputable fact that policy and programs in aging have been based almost entirely on the perceived characteristics of those who are currently elderly. If, as we have maintained, our society will increasingly consist of educated, professional people (with longer life spans), then it is necessary to begin to think about what possible futures might look like from the perspective of our view (undoubtedly wrong in certain respects) of the characteristics of today's younger people. This is a tall and risky order but needs to be attempted if only, as we shall do, with respect to some of its educational implications.

EDUCATIONAL IMPLICATIONS[4]

It is not because we are optimists, or believers in progress and the inevitability of "good" winning out over "bad," or because we have any sense of security in weighing the significances of diverse social trends that we shall note and discuss some recent suggestions and developments. Within several months of each other there appeared two publications. One was *Youth: Transition to Adulthood*, a report of the Panel on Youth of the President's Science Advisory Committee (1973). A major recommendation in this report is that in high school years work and school should be co-equal experiences, that is, that work should not be an after-school or summer experience. During these years the world of work can be as productive of knowledge, factual and conceptual, as sitting in a classroom. What is noteworthy about this recommendation is that it is meant to apply to all students and not only, as in the past, to those destined to be blue or white collar workers. This recommendation, of course, makes no sense unless it reflects the fact that high school students are massively indifferent to their school experiences—a conclusion well documented by Buxton (1973)—as well as the conclusion that work has become problematic for *all* segments of society. The second publication was *Scholarship in Society, a Report on Emerging Roles and Responsibilities of Graduate Education in America* (1973). One of its recommendations for graduate education is no different than what was recommended for high school students, with the additional suggestion that graduate education be made far easier than it now is for those able only to go part-time. And then Boyer (1974), as Chancellor of the State University of New York, has vigorously supported lifelong education and flexibility in educational programming.

What is significant about all these recommendations is not their newness (they are not all that new) but who is presenting them. In each instance they are either policy makers or people in positions of influencing educational policy. When these kinds of people are calling

---

[4] It is our impression that what we have to say in this article about the problematic nature of work for professional people has first been said by social critics, novelists, and artists rather than by social scientists. If there is any question about priority, there can be none about sensitivity and description of the issues. See, for example, DeMott's (1971) slender but powerful book of social comment *Surviving the 70's*, amazingly similar in theme and thrust to what we have earlier presented in this article.

for a realignment between the world of work and school, it is safe to assume that they are reflecting widespread dissatisfaction with both worlds for *all* segments of society.

We have no quarrel with these suggestions except in one respect. *The major thrust of these suggestions implicitly assumes or does not explicitly question that people should choose a single career or that people are and in the future will continue to be satisfied with one career.* The problem these suggestions attack is how to help people make this choice on grounds of more varied experiences in the world of work. One must applaud any suggestion that would make it easier for people of all ages to avail themselves of more education, be it for sheer intellectual pleasure or refinement of existing skills. But if, as we think it increasingly to be the case, people will seek career changes both small and great in degree, then the suggestions above do not get to the heart of the matter.[5] And the heart of the matter, like the structure of the atom, is fantastically complex. After all, we are dealing with attitudes and practices deeply ingrained in our culture and reflected in the substance and structure of education, of our economic system, and of the family. We have said that important changes may be taking place in regards to the concept of the single career and we are now emphasizing the obstacles such changes must encounter. For example, if one looks at children's books—those used in or out of schools—it quickly becomes obvious how directly or indirectly we instill in children the idea of a single career. And if one looks at the "career messages" students receive in high school, it is also obvious that students are asked to think in terms of a single career. It used to be that the college-bound student was expected to choose a single college in which, *of course*, he would spend four years. This is no longer true. Unlike the past when the student who wanted to transfer was made to feel atypical and it was extraordinarily difficult for him to be admitted elsewhere, we now view it more positively and indeed encourage it. It also used to be that the college student who wanted to take a year off, almost regardless of reason, would encounter administrative rules, regulations, and attitudes that seemed based on two assumptions: It should be made difficult for the student, and his motivations should be suspect unless he clearly could prove otherwise.

---

[5] The reader should consult a book *Essays on Career Education* (McClure & Baun 1973). The first paper is by an anthropologist, J. P. Spradley, who raises and discusses the necessity of thinking through the educational and cultural implications of the concept of multiple careers. Twenty-one of the remaining 22 papers (Thomas F. Green, not surprisingly, being the exception) never take up the questions Spradley addresses. When one considers that this book has the imprimatur of the Office of Education, one cannot be enthusiastic about what to expect from renewed interest and funding in career education.

Despite these and similar changes and their implications, the thrust and structure of the college years are to help the student make a life-enduring choice. That this "help" is increasingly experienced by the student as untimely and unreasoned pressure, stemming from the fear of making *the* wrong decision among a welter of possibilities, either goes unrecognized or is interpreted as a reluctance to face up to the realities of life. "They are afraid to grow up"—and indeed many are—but it would be the most ludicrous form of psychologizing to explain the fear exclusively in intrapsychic terms.

If we are correct in our assessment, the concept of lifelong education must deal directly with two questions: How do we prepare children of all ages for thinking about and planning for more than one career?[6] How do we begin to make it more possible for people to change careers without indulging dilettantism and requiring a self-defeating degree of sacrifice? The second question is the more thorny of the two because it so obviously brings to the fore the economic structure of marriage, business, industry, professional work, and education itself. It would be inappropriate for us in this article either to anticipate the many problems that would arise or to attempt to outline schemes by which they could be dealt with. The immediate task has been to suggest that the change process has already begun because the nature of work in our society has made many people dissatisfied and has forced some to actively seek a change. We are not talking about something that may happen but about something that is happening, and we have chosen to emphasize the potential significances of it among the highly educated who will represent an increasing segment of our population.

Ours is a society that prides itself on the ever-expanding opportunities that education provides to more and more segments of the population. These opportunities create and reinforce rising expectations about what to expect over the life span, not only in a material sense but also in terms of level of personal satisfaction. It is our belief that for some time the highly educated, professional person has been aware of a discrepency between what he expected and what he experiences in his work, and that the younger people of today anxiously

---

[6]One of our studies by Fountain (1975) focused on job satisfaction of teachers, who in comparison to other professionals tend to report significantly lower levels of satisfaction. She interviewed most of the teachers in one high school and found a level of job satisfaction higher than was reported in other studies. But she also found that for a surprising number of interviewees teaching was a second or third career, in which respect this school was probably atypical. Their satisfaction was as much a reaction to previously unsatisfying work as it was to what they perceived to be worthy work. We would be very surprised if the students knew the work histories of their teachers.

sense that this is what is in store for them and they have difficulty thinking about a future that will deny expression to their needs, talents, and interests. Young people ordinarily do not worry about aging in its conventional sense, and they do not have a long future perspective. But what many of them do have is a heightened sensitivity to the worthwhileness of how they are "filling in" and will fill in time, and it is our suggestion that how that sensitivity continues to develop is fateful for when and how they become aware of aging in its more conventional sense. Intuitively and inchoately they know that their relationship to their work will be a major factor in their experience of worthwhileness. Their intuitions have a basis in a reality that justifies a dysphoric wariness.

REFERENCES

Boyer, E. Higher education for all, through old age. *New York Times*, April 8, 1974.

Buxton, C. E. *Adolescents in school*. New Haven, Conn.: Yale University Press, 1973.

DeMott, B. *Surviving the 70's*. New York: Dutton, 1971.

Fountain, P. *What teaching does to teachers*. Unpublished doctoral dissertation, Yale University, 1975.

Green, T. *Work, leisure, and the American schools*. New York: Random House, 1968.

Lieberman, V. *Sexual problems in family practice: Why don't physicians refer?* Unpublished master's thesis, Department of Epidemiology and Public Health, Yale University, 1974.

Maynard, J. *Growing up old in the sixties*. New York: Doubleday, 1973.

McClure, L., & Baun, C. (Eds.). *Essays on career education*. Washington, D.C.: U.S. Government Printing Office, 1973.

President's Science Advisory Committee. *Youth: Transition to adulthood*. Washington, D.C.: U.S. Government Printing Office, 1973.

Sarason, S. B. *The creation of settings and the future societies*. San Francisco: Jossey-Bass, 1972.

Sarason, S. B. *The psychological sense of community. Prospects for a community psychology*. San Francisco: Jossey-Bass, 1974.

Scholarship in society, a report on emerging roles and responsibilities of graduate education in America. Princeton, N.J.: Educational Testing Service, 1973.

Spradley, J. P. Career education in cultural perspective. In L. McClure & Baun (Eds.), *Essays on career education*. Washington, D.C.: U.S. Government Printing Office, 1973.

Terkel, S. *Working*. New York: Pantheon, 1974.

8

Career Change: An Autobiographical Fragment

A major, and certainly the most heroic, contribution of Freud was in asserting and demonstrating that his theory was not only for "them," the patients, but for the psychotherapist as well. Just as you do not need one theory for the oxygen atom and another for the helium atom, Freud developed a theory as applicable to one as to another human being. Whatever its shortcomings and distortions, none of its critics has questioned it on the grounds that it is applicable only to "them" and not to "us." The problem is no different when it comes to analysis and discussion of a problem of the culture of which one is part. Concretely, this book is about highly educated, professional people in our society. I am such a person. It would be fiction to write as if I were only talking about "them" and not myself. As I became interested in work, aging, and social change I was inevitably confronted with three major issues. First, I was becoming involved with a set of problems about "them" to which I was far from indifferent or neutral, and even if one made the invalid assumption that their problems were not my problems, we shared a common culture and to that extent I was not an impersonal observer or investigator. Could I under these circurstances maintain sufficient distance to describe, analyze, and understand with some "objectivity" an aspect of social reality? And if sharing a common culture was not problem enough, there was the additional fact of a sizeable age difference between me and many of them. The very fact that I was acutely aware of the implications of this age difference already reflected that we were living in a certain society at a particular time and not in much earlier

S. B. Sarason, "Career Change: An Autobiographical Fragment," Chapter IX in *Work, Aging, and Social Change* (New York: Free Press, 1977). Copyright © 1977 by The Free Press, a Division of Macmillan Publishing Co., Inc. Reprinted with permission.

times or societies where awareness of generational differences would have very different contents. Finally, and crucially, I was grappling with the problems of work, aging, and social change in the most personal ways, and that is for a writer-investigator a blessing and a trap—and a danger for the unsuspecting reader who likes to believe that the author of a book like this is an impersonal conduit of the "real world." Frankly, I was less concerned for the unsuspecting reader than I was for my unsuspecting self, because I did not want to feel that I would end up deceiving myself (too much).

There are no surefire ways of solving these issues, although some people try to do it by resorting to procedures which too often trivialize the problems they are working on or result in misdirected focus or emphasis. These procedures are quite appropriate when there is general agreement that the questions being studied are well formulated and their complexity recognized, so that there is conceptual control against triviality and irrelevance. I am not dealing with questions of this kind, although I believe that in the coming decades they will increasingly force themselves into prominence and thereby gain in sharpness of formulation.

The above is prologue to an autobiographical fragment. Its purpose is less to tell the reader about myself but more to serve as a vehicle to raise questions about career and career change. We are desperately in need of systematic data which are minimally distorted by personal experience and bias, but we need even more the security that such data are being gathered because they will illuminate and not obscure complexities.

1935 was midway in the Great Depression. My father was out of work, and there were times when we did not know if there would be a next meal. Going to college that year would have been an utter impossibility were it not, strangely enough, for the fact that I had had polio and had just undergone corrective surgery. The operation was made possible, first, as a consequence of a letter I had sent to President Franklin D. Roosevelt and, second, through arrangements made by the New Jersey State Rehabilitation Commission. It was the latter agency who paid one-half of my tuition ($150) to a local commuter-type university; the other half was obtained through a university loan to be paid back after I had graduated. If I had been unable to go to college, I would have done nothing; I literally could not have worked.

College was a magnificent experience, intellectually and socially. I had wonderful teachers and made lasting friendships. I was politically active and left wing (Trotskyite) and quite involved in a variety of student organizations. I lacked certainty about many things, one of them being what I would do when I got through college. For the first three years I do not think I gave much thought to the matter. If asked, I would say I probably would go to law school, but that had as much economic reality as a check I would write to erase the national debt. The fact is that I assumed that I would get a job, any job. Law school was not an interest, but it was about the only thing I knew and besides, wouldn't it be nice not to have to look for jobs which didn't exist? There was a business school in the university, but I never gave it a thought. Given our economic plight, my physical limitations, and the "impracticality" of the liberal arts education, I am frank to say that I do not know why I did not major in business.

There were precious few jobs in business, but that was not a factor to me. Those were the days when the first two years of college were largely prescribed in the liberal arts, and I could not get enough of them. The important point is that I saw college as a wonderful interlude, following which I would get a job somewhere, somehow—any job. This was not a depressing thought, because there were millions in the same boat. I had no great expectations, although expecting to get some kind of a job in those days was, I suppose, a form of great expectations. I well remember a long and earnest conversation with a friend who worked during the day and went to school at night. It was in that conversation that we arrived at $35 as the lifelong weekly salary for which we would settle.

I became interested in psychology. In the fall of 1938, with the encouragement of one of my two psychology teachers, I applied to graduate school. Coming from a small, barely accredited commuter college (University of Newark, now the Newark campus of Rutgers), and requiring a fellowship if I was to be in graduate school, and being Jewish, it was no surprise that I was accepted in only one of the fifteen schools to which I applied. As best as I could later figure out, Clark University accepted me with a tuition scholarship ($300) because they were having trouble attracting students, that being the period right after the exodus of Clark's outstanding faculty under the leadership of Walter Hunter, and before the quality rebirth of the department after World War II. If I had been accepted in no place it would have been neither surprising nor depressing. I would have been disappointed but in the same way as when one does not win the weekly lottery. It would have confirmed my belief that we lived in an unjust and inequitable society where "them that has gets more," and "them what has not" looks on. I had my dreams, all quite bourgeois and un-Trotsky-like, but I never allowed myself to take them seriously except as a form of relaxation. I lived at a time of limited opportunity and of concern for having the bare essentials for living. The bright spot was my friends with whom and from whom I learned a great deal.

The one life–one career imperative, as I have discussed it, produced no conflict in me. Before the Clark acceptance I was headed nowhere career-wise. A job, any job, is not a career. I would have been delighted to experience the agonies the imperative produces. I was not even near the situation of many students today: prepared for a career but no opportunity to enter it. Nor was I like today's college graduates who came to college knowing they would need postgraduate training only to find educational doors closed to them. Career-wise I could only go up, sideways, or stand still. I could hardly go downhill.

I do not think it ever occurred to me to consider college irrelevant because it did not prepare me for anything, except for more education which I would have been happy to accept. So when I went to graduate school I was in heaven, and for the same reasons I loved college: the seminars and my new friends. I learned something about the contents of and research in different fields of psychology and concluded that my interests were in "working with people," and that could be in any one of many settings. My interests here were general; neither from within nor without was there pressure to declare a specialty, i.e., to say what kind of psychologist I would be. This is not wholly true because in the second of my three years in graduate school I found myself thinking about what would make me "marketable." I knew that most psychologists were in universities, and that would be my first choice. But getting a degree from Clark at that time was not exactly a door–opener. Besides, war had started in Europe, our draft had begun, the future stability of universities seemed bleak, and I was Jewish. (I always had known about discrimination, but it was in graduate school that I learned about how difficult it was for Jews to obtain university positions, and at Worchester State Hospital there were several truly brilliant Jewish staff psychologists who should have obtained a university position. After the war they received the university recognition they had deserved earlier.) My second choice was clinical psychology which at the time meant getting a job in a state institution or a child guidance clinic. Clinical psychology as we know it today did not exist in those days. Graduate schools did not prepare you to be a clinical psychologist. There was more truth than jest to the statement that if you got a Ph.D. and couldn't get a job, you became a clinical psychologist. To better my chances to get a clinical job, I managed in my last year to obtain extern status in Dr. David Shakow's psychology unit at Worchester State Hospital. For three days each week I attended various meetings, learned about psychological diagnosis and testing, and got the feel for a clinical setting. I learned a lot but did not find testing very interesting, but if that was a way to earn a living, I was willing to do it. What alternatives did I have?

Today's graduate student approaching the end of his training has a specialty, and at a depth far beyond anything I had. In terms of career opportunities, psychology today is a fantastically more differentiated field than it was before World War II. Today's student has a range of choice undreamed of in 1941–1942 when I received my doctorate. He also has a sense of career which I lacked. That is to say, he has a fair idea of where his working career will start and where it might take him over the next decade. If he goes into the university he knows what is expected of him if he is to be promoted up the career ladder. If he is headed for business or industry, or today's diversity of clinical settings, or governmental service, or special research laboratories, or the public schools, or a consulting firm, he has a mental map of how the starting point can lead to a number of end points. The map may be a vague one (and unrealistic for the individual), but it is a map which he knows others have projected and used. He knows that position A can lead to position B which can lead to position C, and so forth. Each job is a rung on a career ladder; each job will involve him in new activities. I had no such sense of career in graduate school. I thought in terms of a job, not a career. How could I think in terms of a career when I did not know the starting point?

I was not without great expectations if you included daydreams. I wanted to be another Freud, or a Henry Murray, or Gordon Allport, or a Kohler—depending on what book I was reading. Or an Itard. Or a J. F. Brown.[1] I wanted to help people and the world change. If there is anything I was clear about, in the gut sense, it was that people were capable of far more than society permitted them to realize, and that included me. I felt I could do great things, if I were given the chance, but I was quite vague about how I would or could do it. I was ambitious, and I knew I wanted to do things which the world and I would take pride in. But it all lacked specificity and direction. I was like a hitchhiker who wanted to be elsewhere than where he was and would take the direction of the first kind driver to pick him up. I was at the same time internally directed and very field-dependent, a strange combination of me and society.

Every value (e.g., autonomy, growth, authenticity) held by today's students was held by me; the big difference resided in the degree to

---

[1] Brown's two major books were atypical for the thirties. In his abnormal text, psychoanalysis was the organizing theory; in his social psychology text, he attempted to bring together Marx, Freud, and the Gestaltists.

which the society encouraged us to hold and act upon these values, as well as providing some of the means to do so. And when I say society, I mean it both in the abstract and in terms of its surrogates, e.g., parents and teachers. When everyone was security and survival-oriented, how could they tell us "to do our own thing," "to realize our *full* potential," to seek "self-actualization," not to compromise with our destiny, or to suppress our dreams. And there were other factors: Hitler, Mussolini, and the Japanese militarists. The war had already started in Europe. On the day I finished collecting data for my dissertation, the Japanese bombed Pearl Harbor.

My first job, obtained in 1942 via a Civil Service test, was at the Southbury Training School in Connecticut for the mentally retarded. It was a brand new and in many ways a drastic departure, philosophically and architecturally, from tradition. It was traditional in that it was in the middle of nowhere—beautiful country but still in the middle of nowhere. Typically, the only thing really expected of me was to do psychological testing. What else did a clinical psychologist do? The fact is that within very broad limits I had carte blanche to do what I wanted. The superintendent was a former educator who used Southbury to give full expression to his heretofore frustrated ambitions as an architect and aesthete. If he were not the old-line ethical person he was, he could have sold the Brooklyn Bridge several times a day, with the purchasers expressing their thanks on bended knees. So Mr. Roselle left me alone. There were no psychiatrists to remind me of status differences and to tell me what I could not do. Herman Yannet, the Medical Director, was a brilliant pediatrician interested primarily in research. He was supportive of whatever I wanted to do. So there I was, in a setting tailor-made for anyone treasuring the values of autonomy, growth, authenticity, and intent on indulging my curiosity. Crucially, Southbury permitted me to act on my belief that people were capable of far more than they and their society realized. The institution contained a population society had written off. I viewed the mentally retarded as I once did the "proletariat." The *meaning* of my work could not be discerned from what I *did* in an overt sense, but it was that meaning that not only powered what I did but made me a happy person. My friends could not understand how I liked working with "those cases" in the middle of nowhere, except for one friend: Esther, my wife-to-be, who in several crucial respects helped (and sometimes bludgeoned) me to move in new directions.

Southbury was the beginning of my career in the sense that for the first time I was able to clarify what I was like, could do, and wanted to do. I knew I was at point *A*, that I wanted to get to point

B, and then *C*, and so forth. I no longer felt like a passive reed not knowing in which direction I would be bent by the next breeze. *I was now in control of my own destiny*, a very un-Skinner-like position, but then again Skinner has never understood the issues of will and freedom in the William James sense which Barrett has recently so pithily described. When I said point *A* and point *B* I was not referring to geographical points, because what I wanted to do and learn could be (could *only* be) found at Southbury. Literally, I was prepared to spend many years there. With Esther's help I had started a number of research projects, we were learning about and practicing psychotherapy, I was being psychoanalyzed, we went to New York to learn Rorschach from Bruno Klopfer, and I thoroughly enjoyed my intrusions into the different aspects of the institution's functioning. Besides, my starting salary was $2280, and I had received increases to $2850! (We did have an apartment on the grounds for $316 a year.)

Although in the middle of nowhere, Southbury gave me intellectual freedom and those conditions in which my values received expression. I was aware that Southbury could spoil me for other and better-paying jobs which began to come along as the armed services began to absorb a good portion of civilian health personnel. Where else could I learn as much and grow as fast? *The fact is that what I was experiencing at Southbury was what the post-World War II generations were taught to want and expect.* It was all right for my generation to want but not to expect such outcomes. I learned one thing at Southbury that I was unprepared for, and which few psychologists (then and now) ever learn. I think it is true that nothing in my experience or education prepared me for what life in a complicated organization was like, especially in a geographically isolated one like Southbury (during a war-time period when cars and gasoline were precious commodities). Suffice to say, such living is somewhere between a blessing and a curse. The nice distinctions between work and non-work simply made no sense. I was at Southbury four years and midway in my stay the Peyton Place–Something Happened social dynamics began to erode the picture of paradise I have previously painted. This does not mean that I seriously thought of leaving, but rather that Esther and I began to feel socially confined and irritated at the ways in which organizational and social craziness intruded into our "work."

Getting a position in a university was not in my plans, because I did not see it as a realistic possibility and not because I had ruled it out. So when the opportunity arose in 1946 to go to Yale, I was pleased and excited. (Unfortunately, I cannot relate in this fragment how this opportunity occurred, but it is quite a story.) This raises an interesting and important question: was the switch from South- bury to Yale a career change or simply another job in a career as a psychologist? Phenomenologically, it was a career change. There was practically no overlap in my responsibilities in the two settings. The people to whom I would relate (e.g., faculty, students) were obviously different in terms of background and function from those of South- bury. At Southbury my working hours were set; at Yale I taught several hours a week, and how to spend the rest of the time was my responsibility. And Yale and Southbury were quite dissimilar on scores of dimensions. Yale was a new world and a new life for me. Yes, I would teach some of the things I had learned at Southbury, and I would continue to do research but in different ways and on different aspects of human functioning. Indeed, I did not have to restrict my research to mental retardation, and I did move in new directions. Therefore, to say that I had taken a new job *as a psycholo- gist,* with the implication that there was significant overlap between the two jobs that did not involve a truly drastic change in how I thought and what I thought about, is to distort my phenomenology to fit pre-existing catagories. I said earlier that it was not until I was at Southbury that I developed a sense of career, i.e., the future began to take shape, and I could begin to see the roads which would lead me to that future. I indicated what that meant, but there was more to it, e.g., getting more psychologists at Southbury, perhaps moving as chief to a better-paying and larger department in another institution, or even becoming head of such an institution (my masochism in those days knew no bounds!). I also toyed with the possibility of shifting to a state mental hospital in which there would be new opportuni- ties to learn and grow—and gain more status and income. If I had gone in any of these directions, the overlap between any of them and Southbury would have been very significant. It would have been a move "up" in a familiar career pattern. Moving to the university was literally a new ballgame with new rules, traditions, functions, turf, and horizons. Soccer and football have a number of things in common not the least of which is speed, agility, physical contact, kicking a ball, etc. But the soccer player has, so to speak, to start all over again when he wants to become a football player, and vice versa. (The one exception, of course, is the soccer player who becomes a place kicker in football—a function so specialized that it is mischievous to say he has become a football player.)

My purpose has not been to draw sharp distinctions but rather to suggest that what conventional thinking often regards as a stage in a career line or pattern—a line of natural ascent—may be phenomenologically the start of a new life or new career. And that is the point: the change may be powered by the desire for a new way of living and thinking, however much one's public label remains the same. I was a psychologist the day I left Southbury, and I was the "same" psychologist when I came to Yale, but the identity of public labels hid the fact that I was seeking rebirth. And here I must relate something which casts a different light over all that I have said so far. It is not only relevant to how one thinks about jobs and careers but also to the issue of candor and the one life–one career imperative.

When Esther and I left the chairman's home in a New Haven suburb, having come to final agreement about the offer and my acceptance, evening had come together with a spring mist which made the blooming dogwoods (in which the area abounds) look unusually heavy. We had about three blocks to walk to the bus. We never took the bus. When we left the chairman's house we said not a word to each other for about a minute, we just walked hand-in-hand. Then, as if by some prearranged signal, we turned to each other and shouted: "We are free!" That utterance was the first time I had allowed myself to say something out loud that reflected vague fears about spending our social lives in an institutional setting, and being intellectually confined by having to focus on a particular patient population. There was a part of me that knew that by coming to Southbury the confines of my career had already been determined: my positions might change, my status and income increase, I would write and do research, and I would try to branch out, but all of this would be as a clinical psychologist in a state institutional setting. When I daydreamed about all the great and wonderful things I would do in my lifetime, the physical setting in which these would be done was at Southbury or one of its different kin. For the first two years at Southbury I enjoyed these daydreams. I was lucky, I had it made! I had *a* career line, thank God. I knew what my life would be like, and I liked the prospect. If anyone had told me that I was uncritically buying the one life–one career imperative, I would have signed his commitment papers. It was after a couple of years, and it was only in part a function of my marriage, that I would have fleeting and disquieting thoughts about what the long-term future looked like. But I never really allowed myself to pursue these thoughts. Where would it get me? Besides, wasn't I learning and doing a lot, and wasn't there a lot more to do? What more did I want? Sure, institutional life and work leave something to be desired, but you have to put these negatives in perspective. I never could bring myself to discuss this openly with anyone, particularly with Esther, who never hesitated to tell me how she regarded institutional living. I resented her putting into words what I feared to let myself think about. Why get upset about what you cannot alter? I saw the future and accommodated to it. So when we walked into freedom upon leaving the chairman's home, masculine me could for the first time acknowledge what I had previously allowed (= required) myself to believe was weakness and irrationality. I had been in prison and thought it was freedom.[2] Relative to any other institution I knew or heard about, I did have freedom at Southbury; relative to Yale it was a concentration camp.

It took more than a year to get used to my new freedom. I felt like a college freshman who, after years of having the school day structured for him, finds himself with a lot of "free time." I began to realize how well planted the work ethic was in me: you go "to work" in the morning and you do "work" until five o'clock and if in that interval you didn't "do" work—the kind of activity that could be filmed and proved you were "working," and that proved to yourself that you hadn't goofed off—you felt and were guilty. You could enjoy this work, there was no law against it, but one of its essential ingredients was that you were satisfying an external criterion of worth. So when I spent evenings and weekends writing, that was "writing," not "working"! I coped well with my guilt, and it helped me understand how much a product of my culture I was. I came to understand that the prime function of a university was to create the conditions for its faculty to learn, change, and grow. Yale existed for *me* and the rest of the faculty. No one bothered me or even suggested that I do this or that. It took me six months to learn that I had "call" on various departmental resources and that the more you claimed "call on" the more it was interpreted that you had an active research program. It could also be interpreted as being pushy and imperialistic but at least it was in a worthy cause!

My experience at Yale was the reverse of that of many of my undergraduate students who left Yale for "the real world." As one student put it: "I bitched and yelled when I was here. It all seemed so irrelevant and theoretical. I couldn't wait to get out. But do I miss this place! I was more myself here." If Yale's primary function is the welfare of its faculty, it is a function only somewhat more exalted than its concern for its undergraduates most of whom understand this only after they have left. I understand freedom not when I lost it, but when I got it. I could write a large volume on universities in general and Yale in particular, and its contents would be far from

---

[2] One of the things I first heard at Southbury, and later used myself was: "After you work with these children for five years you begin to talk like them, after ten years you begin to look like them, and after twenty years you are one of them!" Humor as a way of handling and masking anxiety is as revealing as it is effective.

a paeon of praise, but I would go to lengths to insure that the reader understood that the university is the most refreshing oasis of freedom in our society. It is by no means surprising that as masses of young people streamed into our colleges and universities after World War II they, directly and indirectly, absorbed values and outlooks which were much more those of the university than of the larger society.

The switch to Yale taught me much about myself. First, I had and needed to have a diversity of interests. Diversity of interest and stimulation was essential to my well-being, to the extent that if I felt a lack or waning of either, I would become uneasy. Not only did I have to feel that in the present I had diverse interests and goals, but it was also important that I know in outline the different things I wanted to be involved in and writing about in the future, e.g., five or ten years from now.[3] After thirty years at Yale it is hard for me to recall a day when on the way to the office I did not have the thought: "And what interesting things are going to happen today?" My days were unpredictable and interesting, to an extent I did not dream possible at Southbury. What I am trying to say about my days is not unlike what I experience in writing. When I begin to write I have a pretty good idea of what I want to say, the ideas I want to put into words, and the organization of and interconnections among ideas. But shortly after I begin writing, the ideas and their interconnections begin to change and I end up with something discernibly different from what I initially planned. Writing is a form of exploration full of surprises (and tortures). In fact, I have gained the least in an intellectual sense, and found the task relatively uninteresting, when I was writing up journal articles based on empirical research; by the nature of the task and materials I had to be impersonal and do justice to data "out there." In more discursive writing I was playing with my ideas and I never quite knew where they would take me, where I would take myself.

Another thing I learned about myself—related to the first point as well as to the Southbury experience—was that I did not wish to remain with a particular issue, in research or otherwise, for an indefinite period of time. That is, when I began something new I already knew that there would come a time when I would want to move on to something else. Before moving on, however, I would have to make written sense of what I experienced. I became dimly aware of this when after two years at Yale I felt an internal compulsion to

---

[3] I am alluding here to the fact and denial of mortality, the dynamics of which I will take up in a later chapter.

write a book reflecting what I had done in and learned about the field of mental deficiency. Put in another way: I needed to feel that I would be changing careers every few years or so. The beauty of the university is that it permits and encourages such changes; the obstacles are usually internal and not external.

The two major things I learned about myself—the need for diversity of interest and stimulation and the opportunity to change career directions—are obviously not peculiar to me. One the contrary, as I pointed out in earlier chapters, they were and have increasingly become characteristics of people in our society, particularly those who are highly educated. In myriad ways we have been taught to hunger for new experience, whether it be for a new car, coffee-maker, home, exotic trip, clothes, drug, deodorant, the latest form of self-exploration, movie, or picture book on the new geography of sexual positions. We can scapegoat Madison Avenue for some of this, but it is my belief that Madison Avenue (and American industry) have followed wants as often as they have created them. The hunger for the new, exciting, and rejuvenating experience goes much deeper than Madison Avenue and requires a far more complicated explanation. The hunger goes beyond material things and can be found in our theories about how to raise children and to live our lives, about how we must encounter and confront ourselves so that we experience our protean nature and free ourselves from our procrustean bed. When, after World War II, Dr. Spock's book became the child rearing bible, it was not because parents were truly ignorant of how to keep a child alive and healthy or because pediatricians did not exist or because help and advice from friends and parents were not available, but rather because they thought it contained the psychological formulas insuring two related things: the discovery, nurture, and expression of children's diverse capacities as well as providing the foundation on which they could scan and experience a very diverse world. Implicit in all this was that you had to avoid unduly imposing your tradition and cultural heritage on the child before he or she could comprehend what it was all about. My parents never read Spock but, like so many immigrants, they did not come to this country to recreate for their children the conditions of their own upbringing. If they did not find the streets paved with gold, they did see them as paved with opportunity for their children; and being Jewish made it very likely that the major thoroughfares would be called Learning, Education, Professions. I have discussed this in another autobiographical fragment elsewhere.

None of this, of course, explains my great needs for diversity of stimulation and change. It explains in part my ambition, and I do not want to underestimate what it meant in my early schooling to be regarded as bright and encouraged by teachers to set my sights high. The Great Depression altered my sights, and when early in those years I came down with polio it must have been traumatic in the extreme for my parents. It was traumatic for me but, dialectically, it also created the condition in which fantasy could run riot, and in the two years when the upper part of my body was encased in a brace or cast, with my right arm held extended at shoulder length, I lived through at least a dozen different careers.

Earlier in this book I stressed how the one life–one career imperative can present problems to those who by objective standards are "successful." Before illustrating this in my own life I have to return to the question of what we mean by a career. One could say that coming to Yale meant embarking on a career in the university and that the criteria for judging success were two-fold. First, by virtue of my teaching and research I would be eligible for and achieve promotion to higher academic ranks: assistant professor to associate professor to full professor. If somewhere along this line I was not promoted or given tenure, I could try to go elsewhere and make it at another university, and if this happened I was still meeting the onward and upward criterion. If I made it at a less prestigious university than Yale, I and many others in the field would probably not view the accomplishment without some thought that I was not all that good. (Snobbishness is not in short supply in academia.) But if I made it no place and had to take a position outside the university, I and all others would view it as having failed in my university career. That is to say, the university has criteria by which it decides who is deserving of being a member, and if you don't meet those criteria a career in the university is impossible. Your career has been aborted. Implicit in the conception of a career is that one has "improved" one's status, e.g., objectified by a new title, or more underlings, or more income, or all three. A career is a ladder which has definite, albeit varying, rungs leading to an agreed upon desirable elevation. One climbs the ladder, unless one falls or is pushed off. The length of the ladder varies from one profession to another, as well as in the stability of its construction and in the clarity with which society defines the ladder, but all ladders require climbing. Inherent in the concept of career, from both a subjective and objective perspective, is the onward and upward theme. Over the course of his lifetime an individual may be "doing" the same thing (e.g., a surgeon, psychotherapist), yet if at the same time he has experienced the sense of growth and increased worth he will regard himself as having a successful career, but only if there is some agreement from others.

However, as the mid-life professional related, you can be regarded by others as having a successful career and you may agree with them, even when your excitement and interest have waned or gone. Objectively you are successful; subjectively you are bothered. There can be, and often is, disjunction between how society and the individual define and judge a career. Initially, the individual seeks a career and is prepared to climb the ladder, and there is no disjunction between his and society's definition of a career and the criteria of success. But for many individuals, there comes a time when this conception of career is experienced as confining and an unexpected trap. And if one no longer wants to climb that particular ladder, or if he is already on the roof of the house of success, climbing down or jumping off is dangerous. He has come to see that his conception of what a personal career *should* be differs from what he initially thought and bought.

Now for a personal example. Three years after I came to Yale I initiated research on anxiety in children. I did not have to do any research, but not publishing meant perishing, and dead people do not climb ladders. The problem I chose was of personal interest to me (and I mean *intimately* personal), and I belived it could be studied in a scientific manner. Please note that I said "could" and not should, because the fact is that I always felt uncomfortable with and not very competent in statistics and research design. But it went deeper than that. There was and is a fundamental mismatch between what gives me intellectual satisfaction and the requirements of systematic research. I was only dimly aware of this at the time, or, more likely, I rationalized the dissonance away. This was easy to do because the students who came to work with me were awesomely bright and caught up in the intricacies of statistics and experimental methodology. I learned from them. Within two years I had received a sizeable grant, hired several staff members, and there were usually two or three graduate students who were part of our group. And a marvelously compatible group it was, although quite diverse in talents and personality. We enjoyed and helped each other, and argued loud and long about important football games and politics. By conventional standards, we are very successful: at any one time several studies were in progress; journals, books, and monographs were written; we received increasing recognition; I was promoted to associate and then full professor and other members of the group received good positions My guess is that a good part of whatever reputation I have in psychology is due to the wide recognition the anxiety project received. (I have done much since, but it has not had as wide a reception.)

Early on in the project, however, I became familiar with the mixed blessings of growth and the dubious virtues of progress. Take the dynamics of grant support, for example. It was in the early fifties that the federal government began really to support social science research, especially if it had a mental health theme. In academia it became a sign of professional worth if you received grant support because the project required the approval of an expert committee advisory to the government agency. (It was considered a sign of distinction to be asked to serve in such a capacity.) There was the additional factor that such grant support permitted you to hire the assistance you needed to carry out the project. There was also the consideration that since academic salaries are for nine months, the grant was a way of obtaining a pro-rated summer salary. I am saying explicitly that as in all other areas of human behavior the motivation for seeking support was plural: a combination of selfish and selfless factors. You didn't say this out loud, of course, because it would tarnish the public image of the scientist dedicated *only* to discovery of new knowledge. But you pay a price and that price begins, first, when you take on the responsibility of being an employer in the university, by which I mean that you have a responsibility to produce "results" at the same time that you have a responsibility for the development of your staff: graduate students or post-doctoral staff. The two responsibilities often clash, especially if the grant is for a short period of time and you have to begin getting ready for renewal of the grant. Of the thousands of new grants given during those years (or even today, for that matter) I would bet and give good odds that the number of grantees who did not plan or ask for renewal was not far above some two digit figure. The clash of responsibilities was a minor irritant to me, largely because the great bulk of our early studies came out pretty much as we expected, and I was not in the position of having to worry about whether we could justify a renewal application. Even in those early days I resented the pressure to produce by a certain time. Given my economic background and political persuasion, the thought that *I* was an employer was a source of personal embarrassment. Furthermore, I am one of those people who has difficulty asking anybody to do something for me, especially if I am paying them. My own diagnosis was (and my analyst agreed) that my desire to exploit was far from absent and, given a flourishing and masochistically tinged super-ego, I tend to go to the opposite extreme. As I said, this was not *that* much of a problem in those early days of the project. But the price becomes higher when your project grows in size and scope. Now I had more people to be responsible for and worry about: were they doing all that they could or should? Were *they* getting something which would further their development? When it became time for them to leave the project, would I be able to help them get a good job? If I dropped dead, who would look out for them? I had a wonderful bunch of human beings on the project, and the more I loved them the more worried I became about their future. One additional factor: I do not separate from loved ones easily.

What I have mentioned so far as sources of concern were there, but they really were not strong. Something else began truly to bother me, and it got stronger as this project went on over a twelve-year period. I was becoming a research administrator. I didn't do research, the others did. I no longer had any contact with research "subjects." At our meetings I gave out with my ideas, as did the others, and we would easily come to a consensus about the studies we should be doing. Increasingly, however, these discussions were about what the others wanted to do, and with few exceptions the directions they were taking were fascinating and creative and marvelous for the project. Every now and then at these meetings I would be confronted by the thought that I was not growing. I also found myself bored with discussions of problems of statistics, experimental design, and data analysis. Now, up until an event which took place at a certain moment in one of these meetings, I would have waxed ecstatic if someone had asked me if I liked what I was doing. I would have stilled that small voice in me that articulated doubts, and I would have done so as much to screen out these doubts to myself as to conform to the socially desirable response. How could I tell someone that maybe I was stale, that I had been fleetingly aware for some time that I ought to move on to other problems? How could I explain that it had nothing, absolutely nothing, to do with my friends on the project, and indeed, if it were not for them (and some less selfish reasons) I would like to be dealt out of the game, like yesterday? And how could I get them to comprehend why there was a mismatch between Seymour Sarason—the person, social philosopher, and activist—and Seymour Sarason the professor and researcher? If I had difficulty comprehending, why should I expect others to? In the quiet of the night I knew I was flying under false colors, doing a creditable job but alienated from what I was doing.

My conflict came to a head during a meeting of the group. We were discussing results of two recently completed studies and enjoying the fact that the outcomes were far clearer than we had hoped for. It seemed as if whatever we did confirmed our ideas. At a certain point I heard myself say, quite smugly, "You know, I would be willing to bet that if we filmed high- and low-anxious kids drinking Coca-Cola, we would find significant stylistic differences." At that moment, I knew I was no longer thinking but mechanically grinding out variations on a theme. I knew I had to get out from the person I had fashioned for myself. It was not easy, because what was involved was not only facing the beginning of an end but also the start of a beginning. Beginning of what? As I look back on those days, I can well understand why such a crisis (in its dictionary sense: a turning point for better or for worse) can be devastating and slowly demoralizing for people who are *not* in the university. Bear in mind that what is at stake is radical: severing roots, thinking and doing new things, becoming again a neophyte, putting one's personal and professional security on the line, and there are always the consequences for one's family (and that may include one's parents if they are in one way or another dependent on you). The cogency of these considerations is proportionate to the degree of contemplated change. As a professor, however, in a university like Yale where professors have freedom the limits of which have really never been defined or tested, the crisis was not all that radical: my income and position were assured, and I was in a setting where the untraditional may be frowned upon by some but accepted by most in the name of freedom. After all, the university is a place where you pursue new knowledge and experience, no holds barred, and if that means starting a new life, that's playing by the rules of the game. That does not mean that others drop what they are doing and help you pursue your destiny— just that they do not put obstacles in your way. Yale is as tradition-conscious a university as you will find, sometimes exasperatingly so, but once you have become a tenured member of the faculty the bonds of tradition are surprisingly flexible. You could argue that the criteria by which people are evaluated for tenure insure selection of a tradition-bound faculty, but in my experience that is far from being a valid characterization. My purpose here is not to describe or diagnose Yale (which would mean being expert in the nature of institutional greatness and craziness) but to illuminate the differences between my crisis and those of individuals who do not have the institutional support I had. If my crisis centered around the possibility of leaving the university, then the differences would have disappeared. That was only a fleeting possibility, in large measure because I could not face *that* kind of full-blown crisis. So when I listened to mid-life professionals rationalize why they cannot change their life and career directions, I was sympathetic and considered myself lucky. And when I think what might have happened to me if I had stayed at Southbury or its equivalent, or if I had felt I had no options at Yale and had continued role-playing the dedicated researcher, I shudder. I also feel guilty, much like the survivors of the concentration camps (or wars) feel about those who died. I am aware that I may be overstating the difference, but my experience with mid-life professionals tells me otherwise.

At least three years before I terminated the anxiety project, I thought about what else I might do. Interesting but idle thoughts. How do you start a clinic that would be alternative in conception, function and goals to the usual mental health clinic? How can I demonstrate that mental practices and the mental health industry were woefully inadequate to meeting the dimensions of the problems as *they* defined them? The Yale Psycho-Educational Clinic was being conceived, but there was no reason to believe that there would be a delivery. At that time, Esther was desirous of returning to work as a clinical psychologist and was running up against an insufferable degree of psychiatric preciousness and imperialism. She was unhappy and, therefore, I was unhappy. It is too long a story to tell here, but it was Esther's situation, together with my own and less personal reservations about the organization and thrust of mental health professionals, that finally forced me to begin to take the many steps leading to the creation of the clinic. To separate the creation of the clinic from my relationship to Esther is grossly to distort what happened. In fact, to try to understand what my work means or meant to me without comprehending its functional relationships to Esther and our daughter, Julie, is to miss the point that what I think or do is for them, not in the corny sense of the superior male protecting and providing for his family, but rather as a way of telling them what goes on in my head, i.e., it is a way of telling them about that character they live with. This is one of the major reasons I write. How else can I do it? This may seem to be begging the question: *why* do I have to do it? Regardless of the answer, it concedes the point that my work and relationship to Esther and Julie are not in different quadrants of living.

If the crisis I experienced was less difficult than for people outside the university, I do not take second place to anyone in knowledge of how starting a new life—and that is what the clinic was—can be stressful. Very little in my past experience was relevant for what I wanted to do. Indeed, the greatest intellectual problem was in making sure that I was unloading impedimenta from my clinical training and experience. I had no models to guide me. The first two years had more than their share of crisis. I summed it up in the dedication to my book, *The Culture of the School and the Problem of Change*: "To my wife Esther, and dear friends Murray Levine and Anita Miller for their help and support, particularly during the first two years of the Psycho-Educational Clinic when it was not at all clear whether we would make it."

Was the clinic a new career for me? Can you say a new life in the mold of the same career? You can say it, but it makes no personal sense to me. My office was relocated to the clinic building; I initiated a large set of new relationships outside the university. If you filmed a typical day before and after the clinic started, one would discern little overlap between what I was doing on those days; and if my thoughts could be articulated for those two days the overlap would be even less. Again, I am less interested in sharpening a definition of a career than I am in understanding why people seek change, the degree of it, its effects on life style, and the internal and external obstacles to pursuing change. These considerations are crucial to our sensitivity to the processes of social change because they go beyond global categorizing and behind the facade of conformity to custom. There is a strong tendency, especially among professionals, to see and report themselves in terms of familiar labels and in the light of consistency, even though these may be discrepant with what they are becoming or would like to become. Put in another way: we have so absorbed the one life-one career imperative that we report "career consistency" via labels or categories even though it does not reflect drastic changes in total living. It is like when I get questionnaires from professional societies asking me what kind of a psychologist I am. So, I may say: "I am a clinical psychologist." True and not true. I *was* a clinical psychologist but I no longer *am*. True and not true, because I would fight vehemently if I decided tomorrow to return to clinical work and someone said I could not. Or I could say: "I am a community psychologist" and the same hassles would ensue. The fact is that I resent having to declare myself, to accept a label which does violence to what I was, am, or would like to be. I am more than any one of these things; better yet, I want to be more than any or all of these things. *And that is what I have come to see constitutes the resentment which so many people feel but cannot or fear to articulate.* We are so many things, would like to be so many things, and could in fact be so many things, why must we confine ourselves or why does society confine us to a procrustean career bed?[4] After World War II, at first indirectly and then very directly, this was the message to which several generations of college students were exposed, although society was and still is organized on the one life-one career imperative. Take, for example, the "human-potential" movement which spawned a galaxy of ideas, methods, and gimmicks—and gives every indication of trying to disprove that we live in a finite universe. The very name of the movement is testimony

---

[4]When I say "could in fact be" I mean that literally. We all have our Walter Mitty fantasies, but we also have fantasies of change that are tied more securely to reality.

to the emphasis on what people can be in contrast to what they are, on actualization of self in contrast to accomodation to social norms, on the seeking of change rather than on sustaining continuity, on wholeness in living rather than segmented experience. If the pronouncements of some (not all) of the leaders of the movement reminded one of the biblical prophets proclaiming truth and condemning sin, if the movement took on the features of the Crusades by pronouncing anathema on the infidels (a conforming society) and warring to save the precious soul of man from imprisonment, if the gaudy excesses and flamboyant rhetoric were of Barnum proportions, they nevertheless contained a hard kernel of truth for the thousands upon thousands who came (and keep coming) for insight and change, literally to be rejuvenated: to experience again the lost sensitivity, exuberance, vibrancy, and open-eyed wonder of children. The human potential movement exploded into the public eye in the early sixties, but if one traces the antecedent training and experience of its leaders, one finds many of them coming from one or another of the varieties of psychoanalysis that held center stage for a decade or more after World War II. As I pointed out in earlier chapters, World War II ushered in the Age of Psychology, and the issues of the relationships between what man is and what his potentials are, between what man needs and what society permits, were put squarely on the table and there is no sign they will be removed.

A final autobiographical note. In the interval in which I terminated the anxiety project and began the clinic I made the resolve that the clinic would only take a few years of my life, i.e., that there undoubtedly would come the time when I would and should say "no more." I was not going to fashion my own prison. I was not far off in my estimate of the years I would be involved in the clinic, but I was completely wrong in thinking I could avoid the consequences of growth, success, and new intimate friendships, The clinic involved far more people than the anxiety project, and there were more who were or became my professional peers. By its very nature the clinic would attract and select unconventional people who were seeking to change the direction of their lives. Extricating myself from the clinic was not easy, but it did not result in anything like a major personal crisis. I really quit while I was ahead, and in no small measure that was because I had learned something about myself in ending the anxiety project.

Commentary to
Chapter 9

Until the time I wrote this article, I had been critical of American psychology, but not in as direct a way. I had long been irritated by the sanctimonious scientism of too many psychologists, not all of whom were in the "hard" branches of psychology. Frankly, I sometimes felt ashamed when I heard psychologists speak smugly about their scientific endeavors, as if the label they arrogated to themselves automatically made them more worthy people. They were so clearly nouveau riche *in the scientific community, so desperate to be seen as pure, dedicated, and knowledgeable about the canons of science. Like all social climbers, they confused method with substance, appearance with purpose. They were interested in the history of the particular problem that occupied them and they would talk reverently in vague terms about the history of science, as if one could talk about that independent of social history, and as if there really was a history of science. They looked to a future from a present they could not meaningfully relate to a past. They celebrated their willing isolation from society in order to fathom the laws the knowledge of which would truly serve as the effective basis for dealing with social problems. Their conception of the relation between theory and practice was modeled literally on the most traditional conception of the function of laboratory research.*

None of this would have angered me if not for another of their attitudes—that scientists were more worthy than other people. They would have hooted at this accusation and taken it as proof positive that I was a philistine, but I had seen too many psychologists in too many institutional settings not to know the signs of snobbery and religious orthodoxy. Still another factor impelled me to write this paper (and others that follow), however. For years I had known that psychological theories and research had far more to do with a contrived world than with the real world they were supposed to illuminate, and that, far from being a basis for social action, psychological theory and research were at best an irrelevance and at worst an interference. The more I reviewed the history of psychology in the post–World War II era, the more I concluded that the emperor was naked and quite sick. This article continued my critique of American psychology and is a direct parent of my most recent book Psychology Misdirected: The Psychologist in the Social Order *(1981, 1).*

*Within American psychology there have been surprisingly few
critics of its place and role in the society from which it emerged and
on which it explicitly seeks to have an impact. In writing this paper I
was aware that I was virtually taking on all of psychology. That was
intimidating on many grounds—not the least of which was the erro-
neous perception of myself as a young psychologist who should not
indulge arrogance and hubris. I still needed to grow up, and* then *I
could say what I thought. At that time, however, I was thinking
through and writing* Work, Aging, and Social Change: Professionals
and the One Life–One Career Imperative *(1977, 1). Working on that
book forced me to change my perception of my presumed youth. If
I took my mortality seriously, I had to channel my energies better
into what I thought was most important and would give me the
greatest sense of intellectual satisfaction. I knew I lacked the sheer
knowledge to do full justice to the issues, but I had absolutely no
doubt that the direction in which I was going was the right one for
me and for psychology.*

9

Psychology *To the Finland Station* in *The Heavenly City of the Eighteenth Century Philosophers*

The dedication of a new psychology building raises the question, Dedication to or for what? Is it a reward for a distinguished faculty who needs more space to continue what they have been doing? Is it to have the opportunity to engage in new ventures more sensitive to a perceived and different future? Or is it to live more graciously?—a most understandable, albeit guilt-producing, desire which our society forces us to cloak with the garments of necessity and utilitarianism. If this were a new church we would know how to answer these questions because there would then be no doubt that it symbolizes a millennia-old tradition that will continue to be carried on until the end of earthly time; and its architectural adornments, however plush and lavish, would be justified by its divine mission.

It is tempting to someone like me, who came into psychology shortly before World War II, to regard new psychology buildings with wonder. But in recent years wonder has been tempered by reflection and, finally, submerged by some disturbing thoughts about our capacity to forget (if we ever knew it) that we have been molded by culture which, because it always does its job well, gives us a selective view of the present and a distorted view of the past—in combination they explain why the future (in our individual and collective lives) always surprises us. So if I use this occasion to articulate some doubts about psychology in our culture, it is not because I relish the role of critic but rather because the occasion requires candor and not culturally determined platitudes. Please note that I do not confuse the contents of candor with the truth. This caution, as I hope to show, is at the heart of the matter which, simply put, is that one should be wary of those who profess to possess the truth. Candor has its problems but they are nothing compared to the proclaimed possession of the truth. If we were dedicating a church it would be heresy not to proclaim the possession of the truth. I have the uncomfortable feeling that the field of psychology is viewed by many within it as possessing the truth, i.e., that the field functions in ways and on bases which produce judgments about the worth of its members so that some are seen as superior to others, some more needed than others, some more pure than others. If I am right, we are all the poorer for it. To examine this possibility I shall begin by briefly summarizing two books each of which traces the history of special truths. The first was written by someone who entered and left this world not far from this campus. The second was written by a professor at Cornell (and delivered as lectures at the Yale Law School). Both books have stood the test of time; in part, I think, because the authors could look at the proclaimed truths of others without feeling compelled to proclaim their own. They were not mere reporters or without strong opinions, and they certainly were not indifferent to the scenes of their day. They were too knowledgeable about the consequences of proclaimed truth to present themselves as prophets.

EDMUND WILSON'S *TO THE FINLAND STATION*

Wilson's book (1940) starts with the eighteenth century Vico and ends with Lenin's return from exile in 1917 at the Finland Station in Petrograd. It took almost a century for Vico's writings to be rediscovered (by Michelet). When Lenin, with the aid of the German war government, arrived at the Finland Station he was already an international figure. Vico wrote history, Lenin acted it. Between Vico the writer and Lenin the actor Wilson traces a line of descent that revolves around the relationships and dilemmas of theory and practice. Vico presented a new conception about understanding history and society; Lenin returned to Russia to seize the opportunity to start to refashion the world, in part because he was armed with a legacy of "scientific truths" which he inherited from past generations of thinkers and actors. In 1940 Wilson did not have to carry the story beyond Lenin's arrival. His readers, at least those who were not devout believers in the Soviet religion and its leader's infallibility, did not have to be told what happened over subsequent decades. Hope was replaced by disillusionment. The Inquisition was reborn.

Let us listen to Wilson poetically describe Vico's significance:

> It is strange and stirring to find in the *Scienza Nuova* the modern sociological and anthropological mind waking amid the dusts of a provincial school of jurisprudence of the end of the seventeenth century and speaking through the antiquated machinery of a half-scholastic treatise. Here, before the steady rays of Vico's insight—almost as if we were looking out on the landscape of the Mediterranean itself—we see the fogs that obscure the horizons of the remote reaches of time recede, the cloud-shapes of legend lift. In the shadows there are fewer monsters; the heroes and the gods float away. What we see now are men as we know them alone on the earth we know. The myths that have made us wonder are projections of a human imagination like our own and, if we look for the key inside ourselves and learn how to read them correctly, they will supply us with a record, inaccessible up to now, of the adventures of men like ourselves.
>
> And a record of something more than mere adventures. Human history had hitherto always been written as a series of biographies of great men or as a chronicle of remarkable happenings or as a pageant directed by God. But now we can see that the developments of societies have been affected by their sources, their environments; and that like individual human beings they have passed through regular phases of growth. "The facts of known history," Vico writes, are to be "referred to their primitive origins, divorced from which they have seemed hitherto to possess neither a common basis, nor continuity nor coherence." And: "The nature of things is nothing other than that they come into being at certain times and in certain ways. Wherever the same circumstances are present, the same phenomena arise and no others." And: "In that dark night which shrouds from our eyes the most remote antiquity, a light appears which cannot lead us astray; I speak of this incontestable truth: *the social world is certainly the work of men*; and it follows that one can and should find its principles in the modifications of the human intelligence itself." And: "Governments must be conformable to the nature of the governed; governments are even a result of that nature."

Vico had been influenced by his reading of Francis Bacon and he sought to apply Bacon's science and methods to the study of human history, with the expectation that the laws of history and society could be learned in the same ways that the secrets of the natural world were being exposed. It is not surprising, therefore, that the title of his book published in 1725 was called *Principles of a New Science Dealing with the Nature of Nations, Through Which Are Shown Also New Principles of the Natural Law of Peoples*. For Vico society was an organic whole in terms of which its many parts and characteristics could be comprehended. This is the view that galvanized Michelet, the nineteenth century French historian who "discovered" Vico, and provided him the compass directing his own efforts: "Woe be to him who tries to isolate one department of knowledge from the rest. All science is one: language, literature and history, physics, mathematics and philosophy; subjects which seem the most remote from one another are in reality connected, or rather they all form a single system."

Wilson spends the rest of the book describing the vicissitudes of Vico's and Michelet's formulations: how they changed over the course of decades, in part because of characteristics of individuals who were concerned with the issues, in large part because of dramatic changes and events in western society, and finally because of the attempts to use knowledge about society for the purpose of transforming society. Knowledge led to action at that point where the secrets of society and social change had been discovered—the truth had been revealed—and the methods for grasping and directing the future were seen as logically deduced from and firmly based on these new conceptions. Theory and action were wed, indissolubly so because history had so ordained it. Not surprisingly, a good portion of the book is devoted to Marx, Engels, Lenin, and Trotsky—as well as to a variety of lesser figures who deviated from the "true" conception of history. It would be more correct to say that their deviations were less in the realm of societal analysis than in the methods of social action they thought appropriate to circumstances. For Marx and his descendants there was little choice about method. History had taken care of *that* problem. They had the "hard" data which the "softheads" could not appreciate, or if there was agreement about the hard facts, the softheads did not know how to use them appropriately.

I have not given a fair summary of this book. Wilson's erudition is no less than his incisiveness and both are rivalled by his capacity to give us sensitive, balanced psychological portraits at the same time that he never allows us to lose sight of societal contexts and developments. As one reads the book—particularly if one has read his other writings ranging from the treatment of the Iroquois, the *Patriotic Gore* of the Civil War, the Dead Sea Scrolls, to volumes of essays of literary criticism—one may very well come up with the picture of Wilson conjured up in my own mind: an all-knowing, God-like creature atop a mountain looking down on man and his works, wryly amused at the antics, sympathetic to man's ideals, understanding man's imperfections, and able to live with the knowledge that it is an endless story made up of chapters all of which have the same heading: here we go again! In real life, of course, Wilson was a passionate individual who could take sides. But in his writings he could be amazingly fair because he knew the dangers attendant to the belief that one possessed the truth. As one examines the corpus of his works one can say that he devoted his life to exposing the frailties of truth and truth givers. *To The Finland Station* is one of Wilson's attempts to understand why this happens. He provides a many faceted answer, and I would like now to emphasize one facet: the role and use of the concept of science.

It is, of course, not fortuitous that the title of Vico's book begins with the words: *The Principles of a New Science.* For Vico, as for Michelet, science meant dealing with man and his works without recourse to divine mysteries or to gross oversimplifications or to arbitrary judgments about what was important or unimportant to study. As Michelet said: "Woe unto him who tries to isolate one department of knowledge from the rest ... " Everything about man and his works was of significance and the major task was to see things whole. "All science is one," Michelet says, and he did not shrink from the implications of such a view. It was not that everything was related to everything else but that everything had meaning only when seen in larger contexts. Vico looked upon man and his works in the same revolutionary way as Freud later did upon dreams. For Vico and Michelet science, in contrast to the church, had no rules or rituals—no handed down methods confining thought and action—but was rather like a kindly, tolerant, encouraging parent who emboldens his children to think, experience, explore.

It could hardly be otherwise because, particularly in Michelet's time, the science vs. religion controversy was picking up steam and science represented (among other things) liberation from dogma and superstition. Science was not a set of "correct" rules and methods but a form of permission to tread any path that promised to lead to public knowledge—and knowledge was whole. In the matter of wholeness they were Gestaltists with a vengeance. But as science began to win the battle (institutionally, culturally, technologically) the concept of science began to lose its permissive quality and increasingly took on the characteristic of the stern, authoritarian parent who knows what is right and wrong for himself and his children. Whereas science had been embraced because of its inclusiveness, it subtly became used for purposes of exclusion. If one could label oneself and work as scientific, it conferred legitimacy and thereby defined what was wrong and illegitimate. Departments of knowledge did become separated. The nineteenth century had its own version of the good guys and the bad guys, the hard and the softheaded, the saved and the fallen. Nowhere was this clearer than in the writings of Marx who lost few opportunities to describe his view and work as scientific and those of his opponents as non-scientific. Marx's socialism was "scientific"; his opponents' socialism was "utopian." And didn't Marx and Engels collect and analyze voluminous amounts of data? And didn't Marx attempt to demonstrate the mathematical basis of dialectical materialism? The point is not that Marx did these things—there is nothing wrong or right in collecting data and using mathematics—but that for Marx they automatically conferred a legitimacy to his efforts which permitted him to denigrate those who came to contrary conclusions in other ways—or who simply could not see how his conclusions flowed from his data and methods. He had discovered the truths of past history through scientific means. And, fatefully, these same truths decisively dictated the methods for shaping the future. How you did things was to a very limited degree a matter of choice. By the time Lenin arrived at the Finland Station there was no choice, and for those who thought otherwise it became literally a matter of life and death.

It is obvious, I hope, that my remarks are not directed at science (whatever that might be) but to how people use a concept of science to make judgments about who is in the church of science, who deserves special elevation, what are good or bad things to study, what are good or bad ways of study, what is timelessly "basic," and what is scientifically "pure." It is equally obvious, I assume, that I think psychology may have already arrived at its Finland Station. The analogy may strike some as unfelicitous, and I do not feel compelled to strain at making it work. But it does permit me to remind you of some history which is relevant to what I have said and will allow you to make your own judgments.

In 1886 G. Stanley Hall began planning what turned out to be the *American Journal of Psychology*. The following is from Ross' (1972) recent biography of Hall:

> Hall designed the *Journal* not merely to provide a means of expression for his colleagues but to focus and define the field. As he explained in an introductory editorial, the *Journal* was to be reserved exclusively for "psychological work of a scientific, as distinct from a speculative character." Besides reviews and notes, only "original contributions of a scientific character" would be accepted. What Hall meant by this definition was very much what he had described in his inaugural lecture at Hopkins: "experimental investigations" of the type already common to the new psychology; "inductive studies" in animal instinct, psychogenesis in children, and morbid and anthropological psychology; and lastly, studies in nervous anatomy, physiology, and morphology. "Controversy," he concluded, "so far as possible will be excluded."

Hall's definition of scientific psychology was itself controversial, however. He had limited the *Journal* entirely to empirical studies. Introspective, theoretical psychology of the kind practiced by many of his contemporaries was pointedly excluded. Except for articles of unusual importance, philosophy could presumably enter the *Journal* only as data for psychological studies. Hall also excluded psychical research.

The first issue was entirely devoted to experimental and physiological articles. In his book reviews "Hall set out aggressively to distinguish scientific psychology from its philosophical forebears." And he did this with a vengeance. He did it so well—with such reverence for "modern science [as] the greatest achievement of the human race"— that the journal *Science* considered it "an ornament to American science," and similar views were expressed by others. Psychology had arrived. The revolutionary war within philosophy was for practical purposes over, and the task now was to insure the success of the permanent revolution (a la Trotsky). Ross describes well how Hall was prepared to read out or to exclude the misguided and the fallen from the movement. Those who had armed themselves with brass instruments and organized data—those who could use numbers as well as words—were well protected from those armed only with thought and speculation. It had become an uneven battle. Truth was triumphing. The battalion of psychology was joining forces with the larger army of science, international no less, and nothing short of total victory would be acceptable.

There were some counter revolutionaries, notably William James. For one thing James did not take kindly to Hall's review of psychical research:

> To take sides as positively as you do now and on general philosophic grounds, seems to me a very dangerous and unscientific attitude. . . . I should express the difference between our two positions in the matter, by calling mine a baldly empirical one, and yours, one due to a general theoretic creed. . . . I don't think it exactly fair to make the issue what you make it—one between Science and Superstition.

But as Ross points out, James' objection to the *Journal* "went deeper, so deep in fact that he could not bring himself to express it publicly." Hall had asked James to review for the *Nation* the first issue of the *Journal*. Hall was taken aback when James offered to write a *note*, not a long review. Hall implored him to write a review. James tried but found "all spontaneity has left me for the purpose." On the day before he tried to write the review James in a letter to someone else described Hall as a wonderful creature. Never an articulate conception comes out of him, but instead of it a sort of palpitating influence making all men believe that the way to save their souls psychologically lies through the infinite assimilation of jawbreaking German laboratory-articles. If you try to draw any expressible theoretic conclusion from any of them, he won't hear of it; what you ought to do is to pass on to a lot more of them, and so *in infinitum*.

James was opposed to making the *Journal* "too empirical." Writing to Hall about the initial plans for the *Journal*, James had said:

If I were you I should not insist on too narrow an interpretation of the word psychological, not make it too empirical, but admit a good deal of argumentative matter, if such be forthcoming. . . . I may be able to send you a few little empirical scraps within the year, tho' I'm doing now no experimental work.

What Hall stood for came to characterize or to be the dominant feature of American psychology: an emphasis on method not only for the purposes of arriving at truth but as a criterion for membership in the fraternity.[1] James and Dewey "became" philosophers, less because of any "becoming" dynamics on their part and more because of the way Pope Hall and his cardinals interpreted the relation among method, truth, and salvation. Poor James and Dewey! Fallen from grace because they interested themselves in such devilish themes as religious experience, pragmatism, existentialism, the nature of inquiry, the social contexts of learning, school and society. If psychology had not arrived at its Finland Station, there was no doubt it was building a heavenly city.

CARL BECKER'S *THE HEAVENLY CITY OF THE EIGHTEENTH CENTURY PHILOSOPHERS*

When you read *To The Finland Station* you quickly become aware that you are being treated not only to a creative view of intellectual history but also to a captivating literary style—a master of subject matter and the employment of language. This is somewhat more the case with Becker's book which is more personally written and is graced and laced with warmth, wit, illuminating imagery, and wholesome

---

[1] This has been no less true in British psychology. Indeed, a reading of Liam Hudson's (1972) recent "autobiographical critique of his discipline," *The Cult of the Fact*, suggests that British psychology has managed more than American psychology to retain its "purity" to the present day.

respect—the significance of the last characteristic will become clear at the end of this paper. All of this is by way of saying (again) that a summary of these books is to these books as a verbal description of a gourmet meal is to the meal itself.

At the end of his first lecture Becker (fortunately for me) summarizes his major point:

> If we examine the foundations of their faith, we find that at every turn the *Philosophes* betray their debt to medieval thought without being aware of it. They denounced Christian philosophy, but rather too much, after the manner of those who are but half emancipated from the "super-stitions" they scorn. They had put off the fear of God, but maintained a respectful attitude toward the Deity. They ridiculed the idea that the universe had been created in six days, but still believed it to be a beautifully articulated machine designed by the Supreme Being according to a rational plan as an abiding place for mankind. The Garden of Eden was for them a myth, no doubt, but they looked enviously back to the golden age of Roman virtue, or across the waters to the unspoiled innocence of an Arcadian civilization that flourished in Pennsylvania. They renounced the authority of church and Bible, but exhibited a naive faith in the authority of nature and reason. They scorned metaphysics, but were proud to be called philosophers. They dismantled heaven, somewhat prematurely it seems, since they retained their faith in the immortality of the soul. They courageously discussed atheism, but not before the servants. They defended toleration valiantly, but could with difficulty tolerate priests. They denied that miracles ever happened, but believed in the perfectibility of the human race. We feel that these Philosophers were at once too credulous and too skeptical. They were the victims of common sense. In spite of their rationalism and their humane sympathies, in spite of their aversion to hocus-pocus and enthusiasm and dim perspectives, in spite of their eager skepticism, their engaging cynicism, their brave youthful blasphemies and talk of hanging the last king in the entrails of the last priest—in spite of all of it, there is more of Christian philosophy in the writings of the *Philosophes* than has yet been dreamt of in our histories.
>
> In the following lectures I shall endeavor to elaborate this theme. I shall attempt to show that the underlying preconceptions of eighteenth-century thought were still, allowance made for certain important alterations in the bias, essentially the same as those of the thirteenth century. I shall attempt to show that the *Philosophes* demolished the Heavenly City of St. Augustine only to rebuild it with more up-to-date materials.

And Becker proceeds to do exactly what he promises. He goes on to describe how brute fact and the eighteenth century equivalent of "hard science" were to be the major vehicles for freeing man to attack the task of perfecting man and society.

They were out for the cold facts, out to spoil the game of the mystery-mongers. That species of enthusiasm was indeed to be banned; but only to be replaced by an enthusiasm, however well concealed beneath an outward calm, for the simple truth of things. Knowing beforehand that the truth would make them free, they were on the lookout for a special brand of truth, a truth they could make use of in their business. Some sure instinct warned them that it would be dangerous to know too much, that "to comprehend all is to pardon all." They were too recently emancipated from errors to regard error with detachment, too eager to spread the light to enjoy the indolent luxury of the suspended judgment. Emancipated themselves, they were conscious of a mission to perform, a message to deliver to mankind; and to this messianic enterprise they brought an extraordinary amount of earnest conviction, of devotion, of enthusiasm. We can watch this enthusiasm, this passion for liberty and justice, for truth and humanity, rise and rise throughout the century until it becomes a delirium, until it culminates, in some symbolical sense, in that half admirable, half pathetic spectacle of June 8, 1794, when Citizen Robespierre, with a bouquet in one hand and a torch in the other, inaugurated the new religion of humanity by lighting the conflagration that was to purge the world of ignorance, vice, and folly.

Reason, facts, science—these were the tools that would cut the chains of stifling tradition and provide the basis for the solution of all major human problems. At the end of his lectures Becker cannot resist carrying the story to our own day.

The Russian is most of all like the French Revolution in this, that its leaders, having received the tablets of eternal law, regard the "revolution" not merely as an instrument of political and social reform but much more as the realization of a philosophy of life which being universally valid because it is in harmony with science and history must prevail. For this reason the Russian Revolution like the French Revolution has its dogmas, its ceremonial, its saints. Its dogmas are the theories of Marx interpreted by Lenin. The days which it celebrates are the great days of the Revolution. Its saints are the heroes and martyrs of the communist faith. In the homes of the faithful the portrait of Lenin replaces the sacred icons of the old religion, and every day the humble builders of a new order make pilgrimages to his tomb as formerly they made pilgrimages to holy places.

To put Becker's story in its most simplified form it would go as follows: For most of human history man's capacity to *believe*, to indulge the capacity for *faith*, gave birth to and sustained religion. For the eighteenth century philosopher-scientist the evils of faith and religion were to be supplanted by man's capacity to reason and by reason's most illustrative offspring, science. Man and society were capable of progress and perfection through reason, knowledge, and science. But, Becker points out, the heavenly city of St. Augustine was destroyed and then unwittingly rebuilt on new articles of faith, e.g., obligations to and faith in posterity, knowledge leads to freedom, and love for humanity (the substitute for the love of God).

And when did American Psychology enter the heavenly city? I have already suggested when it came to the Finland Station, armed with SCIENCE, methods, instruments and, of course, the truth. But even at that time the outlines of the heavenly city were not all that murky. It was onward and upwards for the good scientific soldier whose purity and devotion to experimentation would help win the battle against armchair philosophers, religionists, and others of the fallen and misled. To be sure, it would be a slow process but the scientific psychologist had a moral obligation to the saints of science to discharge his task in the most exemplary fashion: to retain his purity despite the frustrations, tedium, loneliness, and failures he would encounter in his laboratory chapel. He himself may not become a saint—nature, the mystery which supplanted religion's God, was not prodigal in the distribution of genius or brilliance—but if he was not on the side of the angels he was at least on the side of the truth. Saint or not, he was working for the betterment of man who, in that distant future of freedom and happiness, would revere those who in small or large measure made it possible. And, finally, just as the devout religionist has no doubt about life after death, the founders of scientific psychology had no doubt about what the end result would be. On the level of rhetoric, at least, the scientific psychologist had *no* doubt. How delightfully religious an attitude!

For illustrative purposes, I would like to suggest that for psychology the doors to the heavenly city were flung wide open with the onset of World War II. Almost overnight psychology was given the opportunity as science and practice to demonstrate how it would combat evil and human misery. Elsewhere (1974) I have described in some detail what happened. Suffice it here to say that "basic" and "applied" psychologists—in the heavenly city some people are more equal than others because some possess more of the truth than others—directed their efforts to saving and protecting our society. And, again almost overnight, with the war's end psychology began to grow in terms of numbers, specialities, scope and ambitions. And who doubted that this was other than progress? If before World War II the American Psychological Association had a couple of thousand members, and two decades after the war it had over thirty thousand members, were not those hard data testifying to progress? And if you wanted basalt-like hard data there were the dizzyingly astronomical expenditures by government for scientific and professional psychology, as well as figures on undergraduate majors and production of Ph.D.s (the doc-torate testifying to a successful communion), and, finally, the increase in journals. How much more evidence was required to prove that every day in every way we were learning more and helping more?

There were, of course, G. Stanley Hall's latter day saints who worried about and fought against the inclusion of the applied psy-chologist in the church of science. They were not opposed to growth and progress but rather to the possibility that these softheaded people —whose methods were impure, whose dedication to "true" science was suspect, who too easily confused facts and beliefs, and who sought equality without having earned it—would vulgarize the true science. As one of them (Samuel Fernberger) said about these strangers, they would "cook the goose that laid the golden eggs." Contained in the metaphor is a view of the past history of scientific psychology—a string of golden eggs—endangered by the present interrupting the march of progress. Like the Hebrew religion which eschews prosely-tizing because of its special truths and mission, the "true" scientists wanted little or no commerce with strangers. Stay pure, keep to the fundamentals of objective method, mine and mind the gold, and pos-terity will bless us for our courage and devotion, because we will have given to posterity the true answers to man's nature and prob-lems.[2] We are and shall be faithful to the commandments of science because they point us to salvation. Thou shalt worship no other God but science. Monotheism was not threatened.

The purists were a minority. Here and there they were able to keep their enclaves pure, but overall the integration between the hard and softheaded came about, not by a supreme court decision but by the pressure of the external society and, fatefully, federal money. Psychology as science and practice were married. Let us bypass the possibility that there are grounds for annulment because they never really slept together. (Each member of the marriage has accused the other of impotence, deceit, and other of man's less endearing attri-butes, sexual or otherwise.) As a collectivity, however, psychology presented itself as miner of scientific gold and as distributors of it to a waiting society. There was hardly a sphere of societal functioning in which psychologists did not become a notable part: business, in-dustry, schools, hospitals, government, the military. Even religious establishments wanted scientifically to select personnel, and were receptive to the use of psychotherapy founded, of course, on basic

---

[2]What I am describing here apparently also happened in the field of "scientific" his-tory. Howard Mumford Jones (1944) wrote beautifully about this in Chapter 3 of his book *Ideas in America*. It is in this chapter that he quotes Heinz Werner approvingly, a quotation and approval that put Werner and Jones in the Vico tradition.

theory and "good" research. When I look back at the past three decades I am impressed, not very positively, with the vast array of solutions psychologists came up with to the problems of individuals, groups, institutions, and the larger society. Just as the basic, hard-headed, scientific psychologist had no doubt where his efforts would lead, so did the softheads have no doubt that they were doing what was in the best interests of society. Despite what the purists feared, the softheads (at least on the level of public utterance) prided themselves on their scientific training and ability to use reason. (Did they not have doctorates which testified to their training in scientific methodology?) There was more than envy in the quip by clinical psychologists that a psychiatrist was a psychotherapist without a Ph.D. And let us not forget that during this period a lot of hardheads ventured out of their laboratories as consultants to diverse settings with problems. At the level of practice you could not tell the hard from the softheads without a scorecard. And now let us listen to Carl Becker talk about the myriads of projects which occupied our intellectual ancestors of the eighteenth century:

> . . . one is reminded of that earnest and amiable and rather futile Abbe de Saint-Pierre, the man "at whom every one laughs, and who is alone serious and without laughter." How industriously this priest labored in the secular vineyard of the Lord! How many "projects" he wrote, helpful hints for the improvement of mankind—"Project for Making Roads Passable in Winter," "Project for the Reform of Begging," "Project for Making Dukes and Peers Useful." And then one day, quite suddenly, so he tells us, "there came into my mind a project which by its great beauty struck me with astonishment. It has occupied all my attention for fifteen days." The result we know: *A Project for Making Peace Perpetual in Europe*!
>
> Well, let us join the others and laugh at the Abbe, but does not his *penchant* for projects remind us of Jefferson, does not his passion for improvement recall Poor Richard? Let us laugh at him, by all means, but be well assured that when we do we are laughing at the eighteenth century, at its preoccupation with human welfare, at its *penchant* for projects. Who, indeed, was not, in this bright springtime of the modern world, making or dreaming of projects? What were most of the scientific academies in France doing but discussing, quarreling about, and having a jolly time over the framing of projects? What was the *Encyclopedie*, what was the Revolution itself? Grand projects, surely. What, indeed (the question stares us in the face), was this enlightened eighteenth century doing, what significance had it in the world anyway if not just this: that with earnest purpose, with endless argument and impassioned propaganda and a few not unhappy tears shed in anticipation of posterity's gratitude, it devoted all its energies to sketching the most naively simple project ever seen for making dukes and peers useful, for opening all roads available to the pursuit of happiness, for

securing the blessings of liberty, equality, and fraternity to all mankind? Maybe this project was less futile than those of the Abbe de Saint-Pierre, maybe it only seems so; but it was at all events inspired by the same ideal— the Christian ideal of service, the humanitarian impulse to set things right.

Up to a few years ago we would have laughed at Becker's description. Incidentally, Becker was not laughing from a stance of modernity and superiority. He was not laughing at all—at least this is my conclusion from reading a collection of his letters (1973). He was not laughing for the same reason that many of us cannot laugh today. Where has our science taken us? Why were our solutions (basic and applied) either grossly wrong or minimally effective? The softheads might respond that their failures reflect the irrelevancy and conceptual bankruptcy of the hardheads: they taught us the truth and life disconfirmed it. The hardheads might say that what happened was predictable from the point when scientific psychology brought into the fold the superficial believers, the willing or unwilling heretics, the do-gooders who by interest and temperament could never learn the difference between a fact and an opinion, between faith and proof, even with scorecards.

There was a brief period, from the end of the sixties to the very early seventies, when the hard and softheads had the equivalent of Pope John's Vatican Council. For that brief period they seemed in agreement that neither of them had had a correct view of the heavenly city. *Mea culpas* were heard around the land. "We have worshipped false Gods! Far from creating a just society, we had contributed to the level of injustice! Far from loving our fellow man we, as individuals and collectivities, had unwittingly reinforced man's inhumanity to man (which includes men's inhumanity to women)! We must exorcise arrogance, social insensitivity, and moral obtuseness from within our personal and scientific selves, as well as from the educational and governmental institutions of which we were part or for which we share responsibility!" It was not quite Mao's cultural revolution during which the universities shut down for two years, but it leaned in that direction and there were some whose moral fervor caused them to regret that it did not fall that way.

But why did so many hard and softheads feel that they had been misled or had misled themselves? The answer is not a simple one but neither is it terribly complex. Most simply put, the answer that was given was: "We had put our faith in a concept of science that said science would provide us with those kinds of truths which would set us free to build the heavenly city. Formulate the problem clearly, study it rigorously and impersonally, find out where your thinking went wrong, reformulate the problem, make your findings public, listen to the criticisms of others, and so on, until the compelling power of the truth overcomes all resistance in others to its recognition and acceptance. The scientific truths will set you free. But science never solves a human or social problem because between scientific truths and their applications to people and society is the realm of values: the shoulds and the oughts. Science and technology did not build and drop the bomb in Hiroshima. That statement omits the fact that *many people first had to say it would be the right thing to do.* Science and technology did not put man into outer space; *people first had to say it was the right thing to do.* When we praise or blame science for its social consequences we are praising or blaming our values, our judgments, the bases upon which we choose to act. When the discoveries of genetics present us with mind boggling possibilities for selective breeding, science cannot tell us how to choose. Between discovery and action are the questions of how shall we live together and by what values. The question is not only what genes we want to pass on but what values we want to pass on. If science can afford to be neutral, we cannot. Living is too important to be left to the scientists and their hard or soft findings."

I would like to believe that William James knew what would happen as a result of psychology's religious faith in science. He was too much like Vico to wish to confine psychology either to certain subject matter or methods. And like Vico he knew well that society is man's creation and man does not create or live by reason alone. He knew that by leaving the house of philosophy psychology was cutting itself off from roots it would some day have to revive. James left Hall at the Finland Station to become a prophet in exile. Although James, like the rest of us, wanted a heavenly city, he did not confuse his view with lasting truth. James sought truth. Hall possessed it. James was concerned with the nature of man and, therefore, himself. Hall was concerned with the nature of science and, therefore, method and data.

James, Wilson, Becker. Of all the things they have in common, one of the most compelling is their capacity *to respect*: to cast scanning curious eyes over man and his works not for the purposes of condemnation, or to erect taboos against trying to understand anyone or anything of the species, or to demonstrate that indeed man was God-like. Nothing about man was foreign to them, except the proclivity to proclaim the truth and to divide people into the fallen and saved. They did not suffer from hubris. Behind this capacity to respect was humbleness in the face of ignorance and mystery. Humbleness is a dangerous and difficult commodity to live with because it does not permit one to confuse education with wisdom, change with progress, the relative with the absolute, and what man should be with the way he is. Socrates never proclaimed the truth, something for which the truth possessors of his day could not forgive him because it would corrupt their young. Hence, he was given hemlock. The need for and the possession of the truth—the need to protect the truth against rival truths—has had an unfortunate tendency to reduce population size. And when it has not been used in this way, it has tended to divide people into superior-inferior, good-evil, fallen-saved, hard-soft categories. You keep the heavenly city a classless society by expelling the unbelievers.

I am not an indifferent eclectic. There are few things about which I do not have strong opinions. I have been and still am capable of proclaiming the truth, although with less joy and certainty than in the past (a tendency I somewhat regret). It is my hypothesis that at different times of one's life one has different favorite stories or jokes which characterize one's dominant stance. My current favorite is about the revered Jewish rabbi in the now non-existent eastern European village. A man in his flock came to him one day and complained long and bitterly about his troubles with his wife. The rabbi listened to the bill of particulars and sympathized with the man's marital plight, and the man left with feelings of satisfaction. The rabbi's wife had been listening intently from behind the door. The next day the man's wife came and she told a tale of woe about what she had to put up with in her husband. The rabbi listened sympathetically and told the woman, as he had her husband, that she was obviously right. The woman left satisfied. The rabbi's wife had also bugged this conversation, and so after the woman left she lit into the rabbi. "First the man comes and you tell him he is right. Then the wife comes and you tell her she is right. What kind of rabbi are you? They can't both be right?" To which the rabbi thoughtfully replied: "You know, you're right too."

BIBLIOGRAPHY

Becker, C. L. *The heavenly city of the eighteenth century philosophers*. New Haven: Yale University Press, 1932.
Becker, C. L. *"What is the good of history?"* Collected letters (Kammen, M., Ed.). Ithaca (N.Y.): Cornell University Press, 1973.
Hudson, L. *The cult of the fact*. New York: Harper Torchbooks, 1972.
Jones, H. M. *Ideas in America*. Cambridge: Harvard University Press, 1944.
Ross, D. *G. Stanley Hall. The psychologist as prophet*. Chicago: University of Chicago Press, 1972.
Sarason, S. B. *The psychological sense of community. Prospects for a community psychology*. San Francisco: Jossey-Bass, 1974.
Wilson, E. *To the Finland Station*. New York: Harcourt, Brace, 1940.

Commentary to
Chapter 10

I am considered someone who helped shape the field of community psychology. I would like to believe that it is true, because the emergence of community psychology implicitly represented a major critique of American psychology: its emphasis on the individual, its lack of interest in theories of institutional and social change, and its inability to confront the nature and role of values (individual, institutional, societal). I say "implicitly represented" because I felt from its earliest days that community psychology had few, if any, roots in American psychology and that the failure to recognize this lack would impoverish the prospects for a viable community psychology. The fact that community psychology had to be invented, so to speak— that it was a direct response by a very small segment of American psychologists to sustained social unrest—spoke volumes about mainstream psychology and psychologists, but those volumes were not being written. Far from critiquing the asocial, ahistorical character of American psychology, far from asking why American psychology was so unprepared to understand, let alone to react to, the 1960s, community psychologists tried valiantly to forge connections between the theories and methodologies of traditional psychology, on the one hand, and the perceived needs and directions of the new field of community psychology, on the other hand. From the very beginning it struck me as ironic that almost all community psychologists saw the field within the narrow context of community mental health. This is not surprising, given that community psychologists had received their training as clinical psychologists. What it meant, however, was that nobody was asking what we mean by community. *Do we mean the bounded geopolitical entities, our role in them, and the way these entities affect our lives? Do we ask what we mean because of the ways these entities have changed in relation to the groups within them and to state and federal government? Are we asking what we mean because, if we want to change communities, we must know their structure power, dynamics, and history? Or do we ask what we mean because we believe that the insidious consequences of the absence of the psychological sense of community are somehow related to (but not necessarily caused by) the changes that are taking place in towns, cities, and regions? Do we (must we) mean all these things? If we do, then community mental health was but one of the different foci that community psychology encompassed. That was the position I took in my 1974 book* The Psychological Sense of Community: Prospects for a Community Psychology. *In that book I began to examine and criticize the increasingly directive role government played in our lives, a role willingly given to government by all kinds of social scientists. For a long time I was among them, but the more I studied the changes in and workings of diverse settings and groups in the community, and the more I began to understand how public policy is formulated and administered, the more I saw stronger and more centralized government as part of the problem, not the solution. The prepotent response to a perceived social problem is to ask that government do something about it. That response signified, among other things, how impoverished and ineffectual the sense of community has become as a source of mutual support and personal stability. I came to judge any public policy in terms of its actual, rather than intended, effects on people's psychological sense of community. I found these policies wanting.*

The hardest task to do well is to take distance from one's time and place. This is especially true for psychologists, because psychology is so ahistorical. As a result, we tend to remain unaware of the degree to which what we think of as right, mutual, and proper is a consequence of a very effective socialization process. This article is a plea for community psychology to adopt a historical stance, to flush out unverbalized assumptions about the field and the society, which, precisely because we have so effectively absorbed them in the socialization process, are as influential as they are unquestioned.

10

Community Psychology and the Anarchist Insight

Modern community psychology was born in the turbulent sixties. Elsewhere (Sarason, 1974), I have discussed its problematic relationship with its parents (clinical psychology and the mental health movement) and more distant ancestors. In relating this history, I deliberately underplayed a factor because I found myself puzzled and uncertain about its significance. More honestly I found myself veering to a position completely at odds with what I had believed, and I felt unable, perhaps unwilling, to pursue the issue. I would like to pursue it here.

When the history of this century is written, there is no doubt that the Great Depression of the thirties will be viewed as a turning point in the nature and organization of our society. Those who did not experience the Great Depression will have difficulty comprehending how it affected the thinking and lives of citizens and leaders of subsequent generations. The most obvious consequence of this cataclysmic period was the degree to which the relation of the individual to the state changed. Before the Great Depression, the rhetoric included "rugged individualism" and "that government is best which rules the least." Just as in the twenties and most of the thirties the national sentiment was that we should steer clear of being drawn into the affairs of the world, it was also widely believed that the Federal government had no business interfering in the affairs of individuals or assuming any responsibility for citizens who for one or another

S. B. Sarason, "Community Psychology and the Anarchist Insight," *American Journal of Community Psychology* 4, no. 3(1976): 243–261. Reprinted with permission of Plenun Publishing Corporation.

reason were unable either to care or to provide for themselves. If you were sick, dependent, and old, it was, of course, too bad, but that was no business of the Federal government. It was a local affair, but even there, citizens and local officialdom were reluctant to render assistance. It was not only that the locality viewed its public wards as failures; so did the public ward view him or herself. It was literally inconceivable to most people that government (local, state, or national) should, as a matter of policy, be concerned with the personal welfare of its citizens, unless, of course, they were a physical or health danger to the surrounding society. But even in these instances, local and state governments had laws seeking reimbursement from the individual or his family. It would be unfair to interpret such laws as symptomatic of a cruel, insensitive society, because we would then be judging it by our present-day outlook. In those days, the bulk of the citizenry regarded it as right and natural that those who "took" from public monies had an obligation to repay, and if they could not, it was only "proper" that the family should be obligated to do so. Ideologically speaking, the government owed its citizens nothing.[1]

The contrast between today and then is enormous. For example we know that there are many students who apply for and receive food stamps, and there are young people whose subsistence comes entirely from public welfare. (In recent months, there has been a minor sort of outcry from public officials about young people from nonpoverty families who take from the public till.) If you talk about this with these and other young people, they tend to see this public assistance as a right due them. Contrast this attitude with what I have been told by public officials responsible for programs for the elderly, i.e., those who lived through the Great Depression. Public officials are stymied by the number of elderly people who will not avail themselves of the Federal food program, even though they need it, because it is a sign of failure to have to "go to the government." Even during the Great Depression, as I can attest from personal experience, fami-

---

[1]There were some exceptions (e.g., the blind) to this stance but they were, to say the least, minimal in scope. They were, so to speak, exceptions which proved the rule. Even as late as the sixth decade of this century, the state of Connecticut had legislation which sought reimbursement to the state from relatives of individuals who were receiving state aid. The interested reader should consult the recent book by Robert and Rosemary Stevens, *Welfare Medicine in America* (1974), which is a veritable gold mine of evidence confirming my central point that entrusting the welfare of people to centralized government (federal, state, or local) is an invitation to social disaster—or, more optimistically, that the evidence supports the maxim that the more things change the more they remain the same.

lies skipped meals, or parents ate less so that their children could eat well, rather than request public assistance.[2]

I am, to this point, not judging the change, but simply underlining the fact that only a few decades ago, the perceived nature of the relationship between the individual and the state was dramatically different from what it is today. Recent generations, of course, judge this change favorably. But it is wrong to say they "judge" because that implies that a conscious choice among alternatives is made. The fact is that the change is so enormous and so pervasively assimilated that most people are not aware that there are alternatives to what seems to them so natural, right, and proper.

The depth of the change is not explainable only by the fact that the Great Depression occurred, although that explains a lot. Throughout our history, there has been a tension between those who viewed the state with suspicion and mistrust and those who wanted it to be strong and influential. There were few, if any, who really trusted centralized authority or viewed it as an unalloyed good. What made the Constitutional Convention such a protracted and difficult affair was the issue of how and to what degree governmental power should be circumscribed, i.e., how to prevent the different branches of government from encroaching on each other and how to prevent them from intruding into the lives of citizens. If the founding fathers were ambivalent about the power of the state, it was because of their experience with and historical knowledge of the tendency of the state to tyrannize and emasculate its citizens. They never regarded the human being as a perfected instrument for good.

Over the past hundred years, this tension picked up steam, and there was a sharpening of positions between those who truly believed that "that government is best which governs the least" and those who urged that more authority be given to the state for the purpose of righting wrongs, eliminating inequalities, and achieving social justice. And who could argue that there were no wrongs, inequalities, and injustice? Few among those who distrusted increased state power would question in the negative. At their best, so to speak, they would assert that social change was a local affair and not the business of the Federal

---

[2] A student of mine, who read this paper, does volunteer work in a facility for elderly people run by a national fraternal order. He reported that a major problem there is convincing the residents to apply for support from Medicare and Medicaid as a way of helping defray the costs of their care. The refusal of many to accede to these requests is largely on the basis that it would be morally wrong for them to do so. The argument that they have a right to these funds, that after contributing to social security over the years they are merely getting back what these programs guaranteed to provide, is not persuasive for some of them.

government. At their worst, they maintained—misextrapolating, as did so many economists and social scientists, from Darwin's and Wallace's theories of evolution—that one should not interfere with nature's wisdom. Among those who favored increasing state power were, to oversimplify, two major groups. There was (and is) that strange amalgam of groups in or near to the Democratic party who, in varying degrees, leaned to greater governmental responsibility for the welfare of people. But even the Democratic party was cautious about any really significant increase in Federal power and responsibility. For example, if one reads the Democratic platform for the 1932 campaign, as well as President Roosevelt's campaign speeches, they are not strikingly dissimilar from the policies of President Hoover and the Republican party. It was not until President Roosevelt neared his inauguration, and the depth and consequences of the social economic disaster were apparent, that he reluctantly and tentatively departed from all that can be subsumed under the ideology of rugged individualism. Big, centralized Federal government came into its own, and the relationship between the state and its citizens were qualitively and quantitatively altered. It was what most people wanted. It was not the case of a Leviathan state imposing its will on a reluctant citizenry. It happened relatively quickly, just as later in the thirties sentiment changed dramatically about United States involvement in world affairs.

The change I am too briefly describing encountered obstacles, particularly in the Supreme Court, which in a number of decisions ruled that the Federal government had exceeded its authority either through procedural improprieties violating individual rights or by improperly intruding into the rights and powers of the states. The point, again, is not to pass judgment, but only to indicate that the quick transition from small to big government, from passive (relatively speaking) to active government, from distant to intrusive government, was not without opposition. In fact, it was the Supreme Court which became a target of criticism, and led President Roosevelt to attempt to enlarge and change its composition. That attempt failed because it was viewed as vesting too much power in the executive. Many of those who supported President Roosevelt's New Deal were concerned, as were the founding fathers, about the consequences of increased power. There was underneath it all, at least in Congress, a distrust of power. But the distrust did not extend to government itself.

The second group, quite heterogeneous, seeking to increase state power, was far more influential than their numbers. I refer to the left-wing groups of the socialist and communist varieties. For those with this ideology, the Great Depression was proof positive of their diagnosis of the internal contradictions of capitalist society and, they assumed, of their proposed cure: a more powerful central state and government based on new economic, political, and organizational considerations. (Especially for the more orthodox Marxists, the ultimate cure was to have the state wither away—a goal symptomatic of an unverbalized, vague attitude of distrust toward state power. As someone once said of the Marxist view of the present and future, "They propose to treat cancer by making it more virulent.")

The impact of the Great Depression is best seen in the 1932 presidential election, when Norman Thomas, the perennial Socialist candidate, received several million votes. In Europe, of course, Mussolini had already demonstrated the success of his brand of the autocratic, centralized state—the railroads were running on time. And, as the decade of the thirties went on, Hitler, of course, was parading the superiority of his National Socialism over the effete Western democracies. There were more than a few in our country who, however much they decried the excesses of Mussolini, Hitler, and Stalin, envied them their power to get things done, i.e., to organize their people and resources for achieving national goals. These dictators anticipated President Kennedy's point in his inaugural address about the virtues of what an individual can do for his country in contrast to what his country can do for him. Stalin, Mussolini, and Hitler knew very well what individuals could do for their country. Indeed, they made no bones about it. They told them what they could do, and most of the people were willing to go along with them. Those who asked the state to leave them alone tended to lead short lives.

The anarchists, another heterogeneous collection of groups, were the exception to what I have been describing. Ironically, insofar as antipathy toward power of the state is concerned, the anarchist ideology is much closer to that of those in our society whom we loosely call conservatives than it is to that of other political groups. Both take a very dim view of the capacity of the state and its governing apparatus to serve the interests of people generally and the individual in particular. But the difference between anarchists and conservatives is a difference that makes a difference. Those we call conservatives (and sometimes, wrongly, reactionaries) accept the necessity of the central state and governing apparatus, albeit reluctantly and with unresolvable ambivalence. The anarchist (e.g., Kropotkin), far from seeing it as a necessity, sees it as an inherently evil force which must be eliminated.

There is a lot of ignorance about anarchism, and it frequently leads to articulated nonsense and a mindlessly smug stance of a superior morality. Let us listen to a paragraph from a chapter, "The

Fragmentation and Cohesion of Society," by a well-known scientist (Orlans, 1971) in a highly touted book, *The Future of the U.S. Government.* The nonsense begins with the words "It is plain. . ."

> The anarchists spirit has been extolled by American businessmen and economists as well as by Goodwin and Kropotkin. Clement Attlee once called the Tories "anarchists in pin-striped trousers"; it is plain that the spirit of anarchy, whether derived from our rural forebears or our robber barons, runs deep in American life. It is a spirit of lawlessness, distrust, and disrespect toward government, and of reliance upon free—that is, unrestrained—individual and corporate enterprise. It is also a spirit of violence which, as one Black Power militant notes, "is as American as cherry pie."

Although he refers to anarchists who eschewed violence, he nevertheless tars them with that characteristic and leads the unwitting reader to believe that violence is the primary basis for the anarchist philosophy. He also manages to confuse the desire for autonomy and community on the part of our "rural forebears" with the spirit of anarchy. Disrespect for the state is evil incarnate! But one should not expect too much from a book devoted to visions of Big Brother Government.[3]

I have no intention here of either describing or justifying anarchism as a social or political ideology or movement. What I wish to do is to state its central insight and examine its consequences for community psychology. I do accept its central insight, even if I cannot accept all its programmatic features. The insight can be put in two statements.

(1) The central state (and its governmental apparatus), by its very nature and dynamics, inevitably becomes a force alien to the interests of its people, and the stronger the state becomes, the more it enslaves people in the sense that they are required, they are forced, to do things they do not want to do; i.e., there is addilution in personal autonomy. The rhetoric of the state is one thing; its actual operations are something else again.

(2) The more powerful the state becomes, the more its people look to it as the fount of initiative and succor, the more is the psychological sense of community diluted. That is to say, the more the lives of people are a consequence of decisions made by Kafkaesque officialdom, the more are they robbed of those communal bonds and responsiblity upon which the sense of rootedness is built.

The problem is not in stating the insight, but in working it through

---

[3] The skeptical reader wishing to pursue the other side of the argument should read Herbert Read's *Anarchy and Order* (1971).

so that it is no longer an abstract truth, or a transient "ah-ha!," but a conscious and concrete aspect of one's thinking about the individual and the state. Insight, as Freud learned through his therapeutic failures, has to contend with resistance, and the latter is far stronger than the former. The working-through process is no easy matter. The task is no less difficult when the insight essentially pits you against the culture, i.e., when by its content it literally forces one to recast one's way of looking at one's relationship to one's world. What you took as right and proper—what you literally never had to think about because you assimiliated the culture so unknowingly and well—now seems improper and wrong.

It would be miraculous if you accepted the insight, because it is like trying to convince you that A is not A. The first line of resistance is to assert that, as stated, the insight is outrageously extreme. The second line of resistance is to agree that there is a kernel of truth to the anarchist insight, but that the problem is less the inherently evil nature of the state than our inability to populate it with the right kind of people—an argument that misses the entire point. The third line of resistance starts with the recognition that one can garner a lot of evidence to support the insight and ends with the rhetorical question: How can one do away with the state? Chaos would follow. Besides, in the real world we know, and which we have every reason to believe will continue to exist, probably with stronger and more centralized national governments, where does fantasy get you? The anarchist insight, today as in the past, is absurdly impractical.

The most that I can hope to do is to discuss the issues in terms of an institution I know best: the university. Before World War II, government had little or nothing to do with the university. Today, it is fair to say, universities, all of them but particularly the private ones, are dependent on the government. That dependency is viewed with anxiety and anger because government cutbacks have exposed the naked fact that the university is no longer autonomous. Its fate is tied to what government decides and what government thinks it needs. So when government decides that career education is important, or that competency-based education is on the road to truth and accountability, or that we need to know more about our criminal injustice system, or that we need new and better ways to test this or that form of biological treatment, or that we will try new ways of delivering this or that form of human service, or that we must expand our knowledge of the aging process—when the government announcements are made, different parts of university administration and faculty begin the frantic process wherein they bend their resources and interests to obtain the grants. The university administration needs the indirect costs to lower deficits and to be able to proclaim to the world how quality of faculty leads to quantity of income; the faculty needs the direct cost either to keep their jobs or those of their assistants and secretaries—or both. Since almost every agency of the government has funds to support university-based research, service, and training, there are few parts of the university that are not in some contractual relationship with government.

I said before that the university "bends" its resources and interests to obtain grants. It is not fortuitous that the entire process of securing government grants has hardly been studied. "Grantsmanship" has become part of our vocabulary, and its connotations have a pejorative flavor much like the use of "Madison Avenue" as an adjective. If sentences in a grant request could be subjected to a lie-detector test, who has doubts about the approximate distribution of scores? The important point, however, is the phenomenology of the grant-writer who puts pencil to paper with the goal of *pleasing* government and the people in his own university, and meeting his own needs for recognition. Yes, I am saying that the process of securing governmental support is inherently corrupting to the university. I am sure there are some exceptions—very few—but I shall assume that a few individuals are little, if at all, corrupted by the process. The large majority, however, are, at best, aware of what is happening to them in the process, or, at worst, convince themselves that they have preserved their morality and autonomy because if they get the money, they have every intention of not taking their written words seriously! And how many people apply for grants not because the activities they will support are central to their lives, but rather because they are acceding to the subtle and not so subtle demands of the modern university culture?

You cannot understand the pervasive way in which government/ university relationships have negatively affected or, if you prefer to avoid value judgments, changed the university unless you understand at least four things. First, the university no longer feels autonomous. One could argue that it never was autonomous, and cite Veblen's classic book (Veblen, 1957) from earlier in this century. My answer is that today the university community assumes it is no longer autonomous; i.e., it *knows* it to a degree and with an anxiety far beyond what was the case in earlier decades, and it knows that its current "patron" is far more formidable and autonomony-emasculating than the business/industrial/aristocratic entrepeneurs of the past. Second, the selectivity of government needs, and the consequent selectivity in what it will support, has changed power and prestige relationships within the university, with the result that certain areas of learning have been weakened and even eliminated. In the world of today, if an academic area is not relevant to governmental needs, its chances of dying are high. The third factor is more subtle and more pervasive: the university *mistrusts* the government because of either its fickleness, its procedures, its restrictions, or its sheer strength. When mistrust, anxiety, anger, and helplessness color a relationship, morality and autonomy are among the first victims. Fourth, the relationships and consequences I am describing cannot be comprehended in psychological terms, i.e., by what we ordinarily mean by psychological theories and concepts. Psychology is not irrelevant, it simply cannot deal with institutional relationships embedded in a particular culture. It takes a sociologist-historian like Robert Nisbet (1971) to deal with these issues, as he has in *The Degradation of the Academic Dogma.*

I am describing the situation today, a time of economic trouble in which the university has discovered how vulnerable its vaunted autonomy is. I stress this new awareness in order to raise the central question: What lessons has the academic community drawn? If you accept the anarchist insight, the answer might go as follows: We allowed ourselves to become dependent under the delusion that the needs of government and the university were identical. We stupidly assumed that despite the vicissitudes of our society, especially its economic Yo-Yo characteristic, it would be in the interests of government to have the university high on the priority list. Far from being concerned about the university as a community, about the ways in which its people and ideas could better resist centrifugal societal forces, we took the one path which would dilute whatever psychological sense of community existed; we made a bargain with the Devil, but, unlike Faust, we did not know it was the Devil. Because we did not examine our values, thinking we knew what they were, we never really faced up to possible alternatives to what we did; we really did not understand the relationship between autonomy and the dynamics of dependency relationships. So what has been the response of the university? Plagued by the memories of the affluent sixties, they want nothing more than, at the least, a return to earlier levels of support, to the establishment of a firmer, stronger relationship! Is it not remarkable that this yearning for the good old days goes side by side with the knowledge that one cannot and should not turn back the social clock? The hallmark of the yoke of an unreflectively assimilated cultural habit is the inability to conceive of alternatives to the perceived order. This desire to maintain the symbiotic relationship is stronger in younger faculty and students, who were born into a society in which it was right and proper that government should take on increasing responsibility for the lives of people and institutions.

But, someone could argue, who is this government you are talking about? Is it not *our* government? Did *we* not vote for it? Can *we* not change it? Is the government a kind of conspiracy against the people, as you seem to suggest? These questions have been raised and discussed again and again in history, political science, economics, and philosophy. My answer will be personal in the sense that it is based on a fair amount of experience with government: Federal, state, local. For the sake of brevity, I shall list the parts of my answer:

(1) By and large, public officials, elected or otherwise, are well-meaning people who believe in justice, fairness, equality, and the power of knowledge. On whatever human quality you judge them, they distribute themselves no differently from the rest of the population. They may, in fact, be skewed slightly more on the positive end.

(2) These same people, part of a large adminstrative or legislative apparatus, charged with the responsibility of making or implementing laws or regulations, inevitably come to see their task in part in relationship to the rest of the apparatus; i.e., their perception of what they could or should do is always colored by considerations of power and competitiveness *within* the apparatus.

(3) Maintaining the size and power of any part of governmental apparatus becomes the overriding objective of those in it. That is to say, in practice, organizational self-interest takes precedence over public interest. This is usually not a conscious or deliberate process, but a consequence of the fact that the agency is constantly competing— and it is constantly competing—for limited resources. Put in another way: the means through which government seeks to implement its relationship to the people dilutes the effectiveness of its efforts.

(4) The administrative apparatus, precisely because it feels that it must maintain itself (if not that it must grow, because to stand still is equivalent to falling behind), invents more and more programs to "do good," justifying thereby its need for increased power and responsibility. Unreflectively and ineluctably, it arrogates to itself the role of guardian of the public weal.

(5) The interaction of the internal struggle for power and resources with the process whereby the apparatus becomes the superior wisdom about what is good for the people and how that good should be given results in arrogance and insensitivity toward all those, within and without, whose ideas clash with the superior wisdom. Slowly but surely, particularly as the range of government responsibility increases, those in government see themselves not only as different from the rest of the society, but also as superior to it. They come to mistrust the very people they purport to represent and serve. Not only do they feel superior to the people, they come to mistrust them. The Watergate stance, mentality, and morality may have been extreme (although I

do not believe it was), but its genotypic characteristics are as old as government itself.

(6) The dynamics of big government obviously rob people of opportunities to solve their problems in their own ways with resources under their face-to-face control, free to assume responsibility for their actions. When those who make decisions are physically and psychologically removed from those whom these decisions are intended to benefit, the sense of community is the first victim.

I know of no description or analysis of the modern state and its governing apparatus that contradicts my own experience. All of them accept the situation as a necessary evil—necessary because they see no viable alternatives. The anarchist insight as an alternative? Ridiculous. Try conceiving, they say, of modern society without a strong, centralized state, let alone without a state at all.

But is it so ridiculous? Is it ridiculous to believe that we can change our accustomed stance in relation to the size, power, and initiative of the state and its governing apparatus? Please note that I am not asking that you go out and advocate the elimination of the state. *I* will do that. What I request is that you reexamine the consequences for your community efforts of what is now our accustomed attitude toward the state. But in order to pursue such a reexamination, it is essential to understand that what would truly be ridiculous would be the failure to see how what we are doing as community psychologists is a function of time, culture, and history. Let me illustrate this by asking you to imagine that we are meeting in 1935, and that all of us are working in the field of mental retardation—it could as well be another field of human service. In the midst of our meeting, someone gets up and makes the following statement: "Why is it that all of you never question the need for our institutions for the mentally retarded to exist? Why is it you are so satisfied with them and keep passing resolutions requesting government to build more of them? And why is it that those of you who work in and administer these institutions, and know full well the inhumanity which exists in them, can't see that nothing will cure the institutional cancer? Why do we need these institutions, forcing some parents to lead lives of guilt because they were told that placing their children in these institutions was the best and most humane thing to do? And why do we place many children in them who are then robbed of the opportunity of being in a natural social community? In fact, is it not possible that all children now in these institutions can be more humanely placed in a variety of alternative community settings, thereby placing the responsiblity on the community? Are our communities so devoid of sensitivity and sympathy—so deficient in the desire to help and share—that we cannot count on them to learn to understand? And if they are inhospitable, are we not in part the cause because we have told them that these handicapped individuals belong in the state institution?" In 1935, our response would have been that this poor individual was either crazy, ignorant in the extreme, or a troublemaker, or all of these. "Ridiculous" would have been considered a charitable adjective to apply to his suggestions. But here we are in 1975, and we are far less sure of our response. Indeed, some of us know that these questions are not crazy at all; i.e., when we place individuals in the care of the government, we are perpetuating two evils: further subverting the interconnectedness within and responsibility of the community, and consigning human beings to a factory specializing in the manufacture of human misery. Hardly a week goes by that some judge does not put a "humane" institution (Federal, state, or local) under the court's jurisdiction until government demonstrates that it has begun to clean its Augean stables. It may be an institution for the retarded, or for criminal offenders, or a state hospital—every type of human service institution is involved—but the story is the same: there is exposure, clamor, scapegoating, and increased expenditures, virtue is proclaimed to have won the day, and sealed-over evil silently triumphs until a few years pass and the cycle begins again. In 1843, Dorothea Dix came before the Massachusetts legislature and described the indescribable conditions in the state's "humane" institutions. Approximately one hundred years later, Dr. Burton Blatt appeared before the same legislature and described exactly the same conditions. And the situation there is no different today! The explanation is a complex one, as I have discussed elsewhere (Sarason, 1974), but a major part of the explanation is that government has a vested interest, economic and political, in maintaining these institutions. Look carefully at state budgets, and you will begin to understand why government cannot seriously entertain alternatives to its inhumane institutions, why it cannot face the possibility that a large part of its apparatus is not necessary, why it reinforces in the minds of people the importance of maintaining these institutions, and why it must present itself as the protector of all those who are handicapped. The state never goes out of business. Its dynamics require it to grow and dominate. The business conglomerate justified its imperialism on the basis of efficiency. Government justifies its expansiveness on the basis of virtue and justice, a far more dangerous explanation because it makes it easy for people to collude in the charade.

And what about the nursing homes which a grateful society has provided for our citizens in their "golden years?" If you want to understand how these death houses came about, go back to the history of governmental legislation and administrative regulations, the political and economic considerations of the policy-makers, and the collusion between government, insurance companies, and the medical profession. The people have been had, as the mass media and the policy-makers tell us each day, as hearing after hearing numbs our sense of outrage and diverts attention from recognizing the obvious: the anarchist insight has received more confirmation than any competing hypothesis. And if you doubt this, wait until the government "rectifies" the nursing-home situation, requiring it, of course, to take more and more direct responsibility, and reducing further the strength of community responsibility which is so essential for any general psychological sense of community. You have seen nothing yet, as future Dorothea Dixes and Burton Blatts will demonstrate.

The usual conservative, after he has inveighed against strong, centralized government, leaves us with pieties which are legitimately open to the charge of "malign neglect." He, together with the liberals, may embrace Federal revenue-sharing as a step in the right direction, unwilling or unable to see that there is little difference between a naked emperor and a naked prince. At its root, the problem is not political but cultural and historical, in the sense that we are imprisoned within a past and a present that make it inordinately difficult for us even to conceive or imagine alternatives to existing modes of state—individual relationships. There is no better instance of this than the unreflective way in which community psychology participated in governmental programs, confusing as it did government-provided and defined "opportunities" with the needs of communities and their peoples to begin to learn for themselves the opportunities and dilemmas of responsive and responsible communal living. As a consequence, for example, community psychology had no relationship or response to programs for the elderly in our communities, programs which were government-initiated in ways ensuring increased isolation of one part of a community from the rest, and setting the stage for the human disaster before us. (It must also be noted that many mental-health professionals were insensitive to the significance—moral, economic, or other—of the transfer of aged state hospital patients to the joys of the nursing home.)

Undoubtedly, you are still puzzled by my failure to tell you what I would do instead of what is being done, or what I would have done instead of what was done. They are basically the same question. What I have learned is that it is not the right question, because the process of answering it substitutes my thinking for your imagination and self-analysis. The question you have to put to yourself is whether, and to what degree, you agree with the anarchist insight. If you agree not at all with the anarchist insight, my answer about action could only make me look more foolish in your eyes. But if you find yourself agreeing with the anarchist insight, if only partially, you, not I, must ask and answer this question: How have my actions been inconsistent with the insight, and, if they have been, how do I begin to become aware of how I can act more consistently in relationship to it? The immediate issue, then, is not about action, but about the nature of one's beliefs, i.e., those culture givens which are part of us, about which we never have had to think, and which define what is right and proper. When you start questioning these cultural givens, you will encounter all kinds of difficulties and resistances, because you will be fighting the recognition that you, that we, have been and are part of the problem.

Elsewhere (Sarason, 1972; Sarason, Grossman, & Zitnay, 1972), my colleagues and I have described two experiences—experiences which led me to my present way of thinking. Both times, I had helped to plan and create a governmental human service facility. Both experiences were highly similar, if not identical, but it was not until the second one that I came to see how the disasters which occurred were completely predictable on the basis of the anarchist insight. No one was evil. There was no conspiracy. What I and a few others came to see was not only that those settings were unnecessary, that they further diluted and robbed people of the psychological sense of community, that they weakened a community's sense of responsibility, but also that the settings were launched on the road leading to the manufacture of human misery. Unwittingly, and with the best of intentions, we colluded with the state and governing apparatus. Despite knowledge and past experience with what happens when the state is given controlling responsibility for people, I could not even conceive of the possibility that the very existence of the state was part of the problem. Not being able to conceive of this possibility meant, of course, that I was another part of the problem. The truth is that I had long read and known about the anarchist insight, but dismissed it as an obvious fantasy. In so dismissing it, I was, of course, confusing the validity of the insight where my actions might have had some influence. Community psychologists, in my experience, are people who would like to change the world. Hopefully, it is a characteristic which will endure. But let us not confuse our personal world with the other one, because if we do, our personal world will not be one we made, but one that was primarily made for us, i.e., we will have complied with what that world says is right, proper, and obvious. Somehow, we have to learn that our accustomed beliefs are literally more a matter of custom than they are the consequences of thinking. We are unaware of this until that point (which may never come) when, for one or another reason, custom loses its believability for us. It is only then that we see that, in a sense, our world had been made for us, and we are now in the process of creating our own. As a consequence, that other world looks radically different than custom had taught us.

REFERENCES

Nisbet, R. *The degradation of the academic dogma.* New York: Basic Books, 1971.

Orlans, H. The fragmentation and cohesion of society. In H. S. Perloff (Ed.), *The future of the U.S. government,* New York: George Braziller, 1971.

Read, H. *Anarchy and order. Essays in politics.* Boston: Beacon Press, 1971.

Sarason, S. B. *The creation of settings and the future societies.* San Francisco: Jossey-Bass, 1972.

Sarason, S. B. *The psychological sense of community. Prospects for a community psychology.* San Francisco: Jossey-Bass, 1974.

Sarason, S. B., Grossman, F. K., & Zitnay, G. *The creation of a community setting.* Syracuse: Syracuse University Press, 1972.

Stevens, R., & Stevens, R. *Welfare medicine in America.* New York: Free Press, 1974.

Veblen, T. *The higher learning in America.* New York: Hill and Wang, 1957 (paperback).

Commentary to
Chapter 11

In this article I call for a divorce between community and clinical psychology. If community psychology remained an appendage of the mental health movement—in terms of theories, methods, and institutional placement—there would be no possibility of broad studies and understanding of communities. This is in no way meant to criticize clinical psychology but simply to recognize its scope, boundaries, and purposes. Clinical psychology is based on a quintessential psychology of the individual, whereas community psychology was created to deal with complexities subsumed under the deceptively simple concept of community. If anything, clinical psychology and the mental health movement should be subsumed under community psychology; that is, the role, targets, and impact of mental health workers and agencies can only be understood in terms of community characteristics. In fact, the limitations, failures, and even catastrophes that characterized the development of community mental health centers (especially but by no means exclusively in their federally sponsored beginnings), are largely explainable by the ignorance and naiveté of mental health workers about community structure, dynamics, social history, and traditions.

I argued long ago that the marriage should not take place. Calling for a divorce was an attempt to stop what I think is now stoppable—community psychology living and getting lost in the house of the mental health movement.

My interest in the concept of networks first appears in this article. I use the concept to illustrate its centrality to community psychology—more correctly, to suggest that the fruitfulness of that concept for theory and practice in community psychology is enormous. In two subsequent books (Sarason, 1977, 3: 1979, 2), I and others describe our involvement in a certain type of network and the consequences of that involvement—still ongoing—for others and for ourselves. Whatever we have experienced confirms my initial opinion that the concepts of networks is extraordinarily revealing when applied to understanding or to trying to influence a community problem. As I argue in this article, action *in the community that is not based on a differentiated conception of networks is likely to misfire or fall far short of the mark.*

Thus, this is an article in which my view of what community psychology is and can be has taken on more substance and direction, at the same time that I see the bright promise of the field dissolving away while it remains imprisoned in the community mental health movement. The reader should not think I am blaming either the shortsightedness of community psychologists or the imperialistic tendencies of the medically dominated community mental health movement. The situation is more long-standing, serious, and general than that. As I say in a footnote in this article:

> I have elsewhere (Sarason, 1974) made the point that the characteristics of American social psychology—in its own ways an individualistic, experiment-worshipping fugitive from the social world in which we live our lives—provided no conceptual framework for either modern clinical psychology or the community mental health field. The absence of social psychology from the confederation is not an act of exclusion on my part but simply the belief that it has little to offer. Again, this is not intended as a way of manifesting any superiority on my part or that of the fields upon which I would base a community psychology. The fact is that when all of us entered the post-World War II era we were conceptually bankrupt before we began. Please remember that bankruptcy does not mean that one is without assets, just that one does not have enought assets to carry on one's business. I am petitioning for a reorganization.

The thrust of that footnote is elaborated in the several articles that follow this one, as well as in my most recent book, Psychology Misdirected: The Psychologist in the Social Order *(1981, 1).*

11

Community, Psychology, Networks, and Mr. Everyman

From the time in the fall of 1961 when the decision was made to create the Yale Psycho-Educational Clinic, we were confronted with a question that came up repeatedly throughout the years the clinic existed. The question we had to face was, Since those of us who were starting the clinic were all traditionally trained clinical psychologists, what consequences would that have on the fact that we had no intention of remaining in traditional clinical roles or providing the usual clinical services? The question came up with regularity because it involved the relationship among our past, present, and future professional identities. It was a threatening question because one way of answering it meant at least a partial severing from our professional and intellectual pasts as well as experiencing the tortures, anxieties, and excitement of starting a new life. This, undoubtedly, is an over-dramatic way of putting it because the truth is that we only dimly sensed, particularly in the early years of the clinic, what was at stake. I think what really happened is that we were fully aware that we were changing fast in terms of accustomed roles and jargon, but we did not comprehend the conceptual implications of these changes.

When a marriage partner comes to the realization that he or she must get a divorce, it sometimes is experienced as a shock, but after a little reflection the person "understands" that the conscious decision had long been building up, that over the years there were symptoms that now were organized into a syndrome about which action had to be taken. I deliberately use the divorce analogy to make three points: Divorce is usually painful; its consequences are

S. B. Sarason, "Community Psychology, Networks, and Mr. Everyman," *American Psychologist* 31, no. 5(May 1976): 317–328. Copyright 1976 by the American Psychological Association, Reprinted by permission.

unpredictable; and once the decision for divorce is made, perception of internal and external reality undergoes radical change. Divorce can be the best thing for the parties concerned, and with the passage of years they may even be able to see this as well as to recognize that a part of each is bound to the other—and a basis for a mutually satisfying friendship emerges. So, in suggesting the divorce of community psychology from the community mental health movement, it is because I have come to believe that it ultimately will have productive consequences for both and, more important,for our society. It is not my intention to polarize, to assert the superiority of one over the other, or, heaven forbid, to plant a flag of possession on new academic turf. If what follows is in a personal vein, it is because I think that it is the best way to convey larger issues. It is apparent, I hope, that in calling for a divorce it is not from the vantage point of a blameless past. If you find divorce an unacceptably or precipitous action, I am willing to compromise with an interlocutory decree.

In the first year of the clinic, our building housed Murray Levine, Michael Kahn, Esther Sarason, and myself. (There was, of course, our secretary, Anita Miller, who was born to the community game.) The title "clinic" is misleading, because whatever we did or hoped to do required that we work in other people's settings. Most of the time Anita was the only person in the building. But the four of us did meet one morning of the week to share our thoughts and plans. Those were difficult meetings. For one thing, we were not clear about what services we could provide. For another, nobody was really asking for our services. Of course, if we had said we were going to provide diagnostic and therapeutic functions, life would have been easy. But the only thing we were clear about was that we did not want to provide these services, not because such services are unimportant or unnecessary—they are vital and socially meaningful—but because they were quintessentially clinical; that is problems had to exist to be brought somewhere for solution. What we wished to do was to figure out ways of preventing problems or, at least, to prevent them from becoming serious or insoluble ones. If we were unclear or even naive about how to think and act in regard to what we might do, we were quite clear and realistic about the manpower problem: Our society did not possess nor would it ever possess the professional resources to deal with troubled individuals. Put another way, as long as we define the problems of individuals in a way so as to require solution by highly trained professionals, the gap between "supply and demand" becomes scandalously greater with time. I suppose I must emphasize the following: I believe that any troubled individual deserves the services of a clinician who is experienced and well trained, and I would argue vehemently against any proposal to reduce the number of clinically trained professionals. At the same time, I would argue just as heatedly against anyone who maintains that we can ever train clinicians in other than minuscule numbers relative to defined needs. In fact, I consider as ignorant, socially irresponsible, and possessed of astigmatic tunnel vision anyone who says that the only way to deal with troubled individuals is through the services of highly educated professionals. In starting the clinic, we were not going to go the clinical route.

So there we were, a small group of clinical psychologists intent on not going the clinical route. As we added staff we gained more clinically trained people (e.g., Ira Goldenberg, Frances Kaplan Grossman, Dennis Cherlin, N. Dickon Reppucci, and Edison Trickett). From what other pool of professionals could we choose? We chose from a familiar pool, but in each case the person was, in varying degrees, eager to depart from the clinical model. In the early years of the clinic I regarded myself as a clinical psychologist venturing forth into new areas, conceptual and geographical. After all, I was intent on helping, and if my goal was to help change settings in some vague way, was it not the case that I had to do this through individuals? In those days the label "community psychologist" was hardly used, and, besides, how would you define it for those who asked? But I was also uncomfortable in saying I was a clinical psychologist because it would mystify people who wanted to know our patient load, where it came from, how we worked, and what our administrative structure was. When I would tell them that we had no patient load, no psychiatric consultants, no social workers, but that some of us worked in schools, neighborhood employment centers, skill centers, regional centers for the mentally retarded, and day care centers, our questioners were both enlightened and mystified. They were enlightened because it sounded as if we were consultants and that is a familiar role (although when we said that that label did not cover our active participation in the affairs of these settings, we could expect a series of questions about what we "really" did and why). They were mystified because many of them knew we were trained clinical psychologists and, understandably, could not square that fact with what we said we were doing.

It is only in retrospect that I can see the earliest events that should have signaled more clearly than they did that I was headed for an identity crisis, that is, that I was beginning to separate myself conceptually and professionally, from clinical psychology and the mental health movement. (The divorce was on its way.) The first signal came the year before the clinic formally opened, when we sought NIMH research support to allow us to study the culture of the school via different ways of being in a helping role in the schools. You well know that grant requests require, and understandably so, that you specify what you are going to do and why and the significance of the outcomes for existing knowledge. We had a variety of intensive experiences in schools, but they were not geared to the problem of understanding the culture of the schools. Essentially, what we proposed was to view the schools as a South Pacific island that we wanted to observe, become participants in its activities, and see where it all took us. This was both a congenial and important approach for me because a decade earlier I had the opportunity to work most intimately with an anthropologist, Thomas Gladwin, and one of the many things I learned from that collaboration (I interpreted the projective tests) was that understanding a community involved bodies of knowledge, concepts, and modes of action quite different from those on which the mental health professions were based (Gladwin & Sarason, 1953). What I contributed to that collaboration was considered valuable, and it may even be that I did illuminate some aspects of the Trukese as individuals. But if you read that monograph, I am sure you will agree that I did not illuminate very much about the Trukese community. After all, if as a clinical psychologist I was interested in what I thought was going on in their heads, it is no wonder that I could not place those heads in the larger social context. Gladwin was interested in the community, and I was interested in the individuals, and we saw the world quite differently, thank God. It was not that one view was better than the other but that they had radically different consequences depending on what one wanted to understand, and increasingly but preconsciously I wanted to understand the social complexity of communities.

We wrote the grant request in an honest way, by which I mean that we recognized the ambiguities of our methodology and conceptual rationale. We wanted to understand schools in order better to see how and at what points they could be changed to prevent the myriad problems for which existing and future manpower were woefully if not scandalously, inadequate. We were site visited by a group of mental health professionals who obviously were troubled by our request. In general they were sympathetic to us, less because they understood what we were about and more because they respected us as clinical psychologists. Try as we might we could not convince them that we were dealing with a complexity that no one truly understood, in which the mental health professions in particular and the social sciences in general had little interest, and the nature of which would have increasing significance for our society. What we were

saying, in effect, was that the mental health professions were parochial and somewhat socially irresponsible; that is, their methods,
theories, and focuses were too acultural and individually oriented.
Our grant request was tabled, and we were asked to rewrite and re-
submit it. And so we did. And we had another site visit. And we
went through the same discussion. And our grant request was denied.
In my more charitable moments I could entertain the possibility that
they were right for the wrong reasons. The point of all this is that we
and they were thinking in radically different ways. They were thinking in the context of theories of and practices about individuals while
we, superficially to be sure, were thinking in terms of intrasystem dynamics, power-political characteristics, social history and the nature
of tradition.

Another event that heightened my developing identity crisis was
a growing tendency on my part to view the development of the clinic
from a community-ecological perspective rather than from an indi-
vidual-clinical perspective. This development was deceptively personal
and initiated by this question: How would I explain that two years
after the clinic started our building housed about 20 people engaged
in a variety of ways in diverse settings in our part of the state? Whereas
in the first year the clinic was a lonely place populated by a handful
of people worried about survival, within two years it was overpopu-
lated with people, each of whom was dividing his or her time in at
least two community settings. The question I asked myself had surprisingly little to do with value judgments. Of course, I thought this
growth was a good thing, but that was a very minor stimulus for the
question. (I knew that whatever we did would be in the record and
that whatever judgments people would make they would make.) The
major stimulus was a gnawing dissatisfaction with the answers that
others spontaneously gave, that is, answers centering around my
personality and ideas. It was not undue modesty on my part if I felt
the answers to be typically clinical or individualistic and, therefore,
misleadingly incomplete—not wrong but incomplete in an instructive
way. For example, very few people put weight in their answers on
the fact that I was a full professor when the clinic started. Statistically speaking, the chances of a nontenured faculty person being
"allowed" to start such a venture—at Yale or any other university—
and to have it grow rather quickly are small indeed. Wrapped up in
this fact are a set of considerations rooted in the traditions, history,
organization, and values of the American university that are independent of individuals and personalities and that are the warp and
woof in which faculty are embedded, developed, and changed. It is
understandable if we put undue weight on individuals, because we

literally can "see" and interact with them. In that sense we cannot see the social fabric in which the individual is imbedded, and, therefore, we are prone to misevaluate its significance for what we are trying to explain. And the more clinical we are in our thinking and actions, the less we see the larger picture or the social fabric. The individual tends to be figure and all else ground, and we are not even aware that there is a ground. And the kind of ground I am talking about can never be seen; it has to be conceptualized, and the basis for the conceptualization is in fields other than psychology. At the very least, they are conceptualizations that can never come out of clinical psychology or the community mental health movement.

A second factor that the usual explanation ignored consists of two "variables." The first is that Connecticut is a small place; that is, one can rather easily see and know the state. It is graspable in an experimental sense. You can know it in a way that you will never know New York State if you live in New York City or Syracuse or Buffalo. The second variable that people overlooked was that I had lived and worked in Connecticut since 1942, part of the time in a state institution in a rural area, and the rest of the time in and around New Haven. If you live in a small state for almost two decades—in roles requiring one to have all kinds of commerce with individuals and agencies near and far (although nothing and no one is "far" in Connecticut)—the chances are high that you are part of or know about scores of "networks" of people and agencies. It was this kind of knowledge that was important, if not crucial, in the creation and quick growth of the clinic.

Geographical size, work roles, status, institutions and their traditions, and age—awareness of these and similar factors increasingly forced me to see the difference between clinical-type or personality-type explanations, on the one hand, and what I will loosely call a community-ecological explanation, on the other hand. I must reiterate that these are not *inherently* antithetical polarities, especially in regard to the type of question I was asking. But it is unfortunately the case that in practice they emerge as polarities, and my experience has impressed upon me the limitations of the clinical mode of thinking rather than the community-ecological one.

Because the distinction I am trying to make is so crucial and can easily be misinterpreted, I ask you to consider how clinical psychology and the community mental health movement have reacted to the work of Roger Barker and his colleagues (e.g., Barker, 1963b; Barker, 1968; Barker & Gump, 1964; Barker & Wright, 1951). One way of putting it is: How can you react to what you do not know? (This point has also been made by James Kelly, 1975, in his review of the recent book by Barker and Schoggen, 1973.) If those in the movement have known about it—and examination after examination of relevant bibliographies suggests they do not—they obviously see no relevance for it in their work. This reaction is not hard to understand because the studies by Barker and his colleagues of a small midwestern community have by theory and design little or no focus on individuals, their psyches and problems. Their focus has been on collectivities, behavior settings, physical environments, ecological interrelationships, and the like. If, for example, you were to read one of their books devoted only to one boy's day (Barker & Wright, 1951), you are likely to be overwhelmed by the details, all uninterpreted, and you may end up puzzled by what the point of it all is, especially if you are a clinical psychologist or even a community mental health professional. In fact, most of their reports are in the form of compendia of descriptions and analyses that are difficult for anyone to follow or to digest. But what makes it so difficult for the psychological reader is not only the form of their presentation but the absense of what we ordinarily call psychological data. We are so used to seeing individuals and fathoming what is going on in their heads that we are unable even to conceive that there are other ways of viewing these situations. For example, in 1963 Barker delivered the Kurt Lewin Memorial Award Address in Philadelphia. Most of us have been to similar meetings, and when we have talked about them it has been in purely psychological terms: the kind of person being honored, his reaction, style, and content of address, our response, audience reaction, etc. Let us now listen to what Barker (1963a) said:

It is not often that a lecturer can present to his audience an example of his phenomena, whole and functioning in situ—not merely with a demonstration, a description, a preserved specimen, a picture, or a diagram of it. I am in the fortunate position of being able to give you, so to speak, a real behavior setting.

If you will change your attention from me to the next most inclusive, bounded unit, to the assembly of people, behavior episodes, and objects before you, you will see a behavior setting. It has the following structural attributes which you can observe directly:

1. It has a space-time locus: 3:00–3:50 p.m., September 2, 1963, Clover Room, Bellevue-Stratford Hotel, Philadelphia, Pennsylvania.
2. It is composed of a variety of interior entities and events: of people, objects (chairs, walls, a microphone, paper), behavior (lecturing, listening, sitting), and other processes (air circulation, sound amplification).
3. Its widely different components form a bounded pattern that is

     easily discriminated from the pattern on the outside of the
     boundary.

4. Its component parts are obviously not a random arrangement of
   independent classes of entities; if they were, how surprising, that
   all the chairs are in the same position with respect to the podium,
   that all members of the audience happen to come to rest upon
   chairs, and that the lights are not helter-skelter from floor to ceiling,
   for example.

5. The entity before you is a part of a nesting structure; its components (e.g., the chairs and people) have parts; and the setting,
   itself, is contained within a more comprehensive unit, the Bellevue-
   Stratford Hotel.

6. This unit is objective in the sense that it exists independently of
   anyone's perception of it, qua unit. (pp. 26–27)

Barker was illustrating his central concept of a behavior setting: a
naturally occuring unit having physical, behavioral, and temporal pro-
perties, and revealing a variety of complex interrelationships among
its parts. That is to say, there is a way of looking at a behavior setting that is illuminating independent of individual personalities. Someone might ask: Illuminating of what? I could answer by saying that
at the very least Barker's approach reminds us, and we always need
this reminding, that our accustomed ways of reacting to and conceptualizing about familiar situations are no more than that: *accustomed*
ways. There *are* other ways. But another part of the answer is that
Barker's overarching goal is to look at and describe a total community: its parts, interrelatedness, structure, ecological balances, and
processes. What for most of us is amorphous ground (the community)
is figure for Barker. If Barker ever wanted to waste time answering
the question, Why did our clinic grow so quickly? his answer would
be radically different than the ones ordinarily given.

    I have not talked about Barker and his work of several decades in
one American and one British town because I am convinced that he
has provided us with the most productive conceptual basis for a community psychology. I am not so convinced, although the recent articles by Price (1974) and Price and Blashfield (1975) do indicate the
fruitfulness of Barker's work for community psychology. The significance of Barker's work is fourfold. He did take on the awesome
task of studying a community. He has provided us with fresh insights
about familiar settings, for example, schools. And, not surprisingly
for someone who is in the Gestalt tradition, he has emphasized interrelatedness. Lastly, the theoretical and empirical traditions (ecology,
Gestalt psychology) which are the underpinnings of his work are not
those of the community mental health movement, a fact that when

pursued exposes the flimsy and parochial underpinnings of the latter. In Sarason (1974) I devote several chapters to the social-historical context which more or less guaranteed that the conceptual base for the emerging community mental health movement would be at best disastrously parochial and at worse conceptually bankrupt. Like it or not, modern clinical psychology and psychiatry—and their off-spring, community mental health—arose as rather quick responses to social needs (and government funding) and that type of situation is rarely conducive to dispassionate reflection, planning and decision making. But more of this later.

What I propose to do now is to elaborate on a concept I mentioned earlier and have come to see as a crucial one for a community psychology that purports either to understand or to help change aspects of community functioning. The concept is that of the *network*. Initially at least, it appears simple enough, and it is explicitly or implicitly used by us in our daily lives as well as formally in a variety of disciplines. If the significance of the concept of networks was forced upon me by my reflections on the growth of the clinic and its varied activities, it is another example of how we conspire with life to re-invent the wheel. Ironically, it is a concept central to the thinking and practice of clinical psychologists who always see their clients as embedded in a network of interpersonal relationships, and the over-arching goal of practice is in some way or other either to use the net-work for therapeutic purposes or to change the quality and quantity of relationships within the network. But when mental health profes-sionals enlarged their activities to include communities, they were utterly unprepared to deal with the fact that a community is, among other things, comprised of related and unrelated networks of relation-ships, each of which can be ordered along a number of dimensions, for example, vocational, religious, political, recreational, neighbor-hood, charitable, educational. I am not restricting the concept of net-work to organized or formal groupings that by custom, law, or choice bring its members into relationship with each other even though that may not require or entail face-to-face contact or any contact at all. For example, as a member of the American Psychological Association I actually know a minuscule number of its thousands of members. But I know who those thousands are (there is a directory), where they live, what their proclaimed interests are, and a few of their demo-graphic characteristics. When I get mail from the APA, I know they are getting the same mail. When I pay dues, they pay dues. I know some of the journals some of them read. I know who participates in the different activities and functions of the association. So when I say that I am a member of the APA, I am saying that I am a member of a very large network, most members of which I do not personally know but with all of whom I can be in contact with if I so desire. If, for example, I were to take a 5% random sample of the APA and write each person a letter beginning with the phrase, "As a fellow member of the APA I am writing to seek your help in disbanding the organization," I can assume that each of the recipients would not question my right "to call upon" them, although they may have doubts about my personal stability. Ordinarily, neither I nor they would think about ourselves as part of a network—each of us thinks of himself as a member of a large, impersonal collectivity that can do things for us as individuals—but it takes the kind of a letter I would write to remind us that we do things for each other, at the very least we can "call upon" each other. The truth is that if I wanted to achieve my goal I would never write to a random sample of the APA. Some people in the network are more influential than others in the sense that if they take a stance they can garner more support than others who may hold the same position. My task is to find out who these people are and which of them may respond congenially to my plea for support. The point is that however I proceed, I am assuming that I feel I have a right to proceed and that those whom I will contact will perceive this contact as right and proper; that is, I can call on them for knowledge and support just as they can call on me.

But now imagine that I have chosen a 5% random sample of the American Psychiatric Association and I write to them saying, "I am a member of the American Psychological Association and I am writing to secure your support for the disbanding of the American Psychiatric Association." The prepotent response would be "Who the hell are you to contact me about such an outrageous suggestion?" I am not in their network, and I have no warrant to call on them for help. I am an outsider. But am I an outsider? I do know a number of psychiatrists. We are part of a network independent of all other networks in which we are embedded.[1] How do I use that network to find out how I should go about locating people in "the other APA" who may be congenial to my purposes? The psychologist-psychiatrist network of which I am a part extends over a wide geographical area, but relatively speak-

---

[1] There is a real question about whether *any* network is independent of all other networks. That is to say, however stringently one defines a network, I think it is possible to show that each person in that network is part of another network, and in that sense one network is not independent of all others. When I have taken pencil to paper to map out the networks of actual people of widely different statuses in the community, I could in each case demonstrate that each person could, if he or she wanted, relate to any other network I could dream up.

ing it is very small. Are there other networks of which I am a part or to which I can potentially relate that can provide me with more knowledge and potential support? The answer, of course, is yes. If it were my major passion in life, I could tap scores of, if not countless, existing networks in order to gain knowledge and support from within and without the American Psychiatric Association. All of this, I presume, is obvious enough. *What is not so obvious, however, is that in the process of pursuing my goal I very likely will have become part of new and existing networks.*

But why use the term *network*? Would not *relations* or *interrelationships* serve as well? Or *contacts*? The difficulty with these terms is that in ordinary parlance they refer to an *actual* connection among two or more people whereas the term network includes such connections and in addition emphasizes that they are an extremely small sample of connections potentially available to us. The different visual pictures that get conjured up in our minds when we use the terms network and relationships reflect the kind of differences I am trying to convey. A further advantage of the term network, as I used it in regard to my membership in "our" APA, is that it forces on us the awareness that we are part of many networks, in each of which we have "call" upon others whether or not we know them in the sense of actually having had some sort of commerce with them. In any one network a wide discrepancy usually exists between the number of people potentially available to us and the number we actually know.

Just as I was writing the above paragraph a student came into my office. He is in a seminar that Dick Repucci and I are teaching entitled "Policy and Management Issues in Human Services Institutions." The students have been divided into four groups, each of which is devoted to a different problem they are to investigate. Each group must write a sizable report. This student is part of the group working on deinstitutionalization.

Him: Our group wants to interview state senator——
           Do you know her?
Me: No.
Him: Do you know anybody at Yale who knows her?
Me: I assume, knowing where she lives, that there are a number of Yale
           people who know her. But at the moment I can't think of anyone
           who knows her and would be willing to run interference for you.
           I could call her up, but God knows how many days it would take
           for us to connect. And even if we connected I am not sure she
           would go out of her way to make herself available to your group in
           the next few days.

As he left the office and I began again to think about networks, it suddenly hit me that sitting in my outer office, was of course, Anita Miller, whose father is very much a part of a state political network of which state senator ___ is a member. Anita and I are "related," but if I had not at that moment been thinking about differentiating between a network and a relationship, I would not have "seen" Anita as having easy access to a network by no means easily available to me. And that is the point: It is "natural" to think of people with whom we interact in terms of relationship. It is not natural to see them as part of numerous networks. You can see people. You cannot see networks.

If you begin to apply the concept of the network to a community, it becomes immediately apparent that a community is comprised of networks countless in numbers and probably countless in degree of interconnectedness. The traditional bases for describing and understanding a community—social class, economic, legal, religious, political, governmental, etc.—have obviously been productive, and it is not my intention in any way to underplay their importance. Indeed, it is my opinion that we have not used such variables in the most productive ways precisely because we tend not to view or understand them in their interrelatedness. I venture the hypothesis that if we were to begin to view the community in terms of networks we would begin to get a better picture of this interrelatedness. At the very least, we would have to confront more realistically than we have that a community is impressively, if not overwhelmingly, complex and that our traditional ways of thinking about and dealing with it have not taken this complexity into account. It would also become apparent that the view of the community which has powered the community mental health movement is parochial, distorted, and mischievous. Fairness requires that I say that this is only somewhat less true for other psychologists who proclaim a community orientation.

I did not introduce the concept of networks for theoretical or propagandistic purposes. I have no desire to push or sell the concept, and I would be the first to confess to bewilderment at how systematically to apply it to better understand a contemporary community. Certainly, one of my purposes was to make the point that if we arrogate to ourselves the title "community psychologist" or the characteristic of a "community orientation" we should at least have the humility to confess that we hardly understand how the inhabitants of a community are actually or potentially interrelated. When I see clinical psychologists and others in the community mental health movement smugly proud of their community orientation and unbothered by the superficiality of their knowledge of what that community consists of, how it is organized, its truly dynamic processes its interrelatedness—utterly unaware that their presumed focus (the community) cannot be comprehended in terms of the theories and practices of the movement, and their minds uncluttered by the knowledge that when they center their attention on this or that group or this or that setting they are confusing the part with the whole to which the adjective *community* gives priority—I react not with anger or criticism but with sympathy because I made most of the mistakes they are making. Some of us at the Psycho-Educational Clinic focused on schools, and because schools were in the community, that, we thought, made us community psychologists. Some devoted a major part of their time to starting programs for and with the community action agency. And there were others who literally created new community agencies on a scale or degree of involvement in the community that was, relatively speaking, on the galactic end. But, queried a small voice, are there not a lot of people who are not psychologists who do what you do? Are they community psychologists? To which the big voice replied: These other people, like us, are trying to better understand or to conceptualize more fruitfully how things are. Do you mean, said the small voice, that doing what you are doing in these different places is furthering your understanding of a community? It seems to me that it furthers your understanding of these different places, but it is not clear how it furthers your understanding of the community in which they exist. Is it possible, continued the voice, that you use the word *community* the way people use the word *personality*; that is, it stands for something important and complicated, but you don't deal with it in its complexity, you deal with its parts and wrongly assume that you understand the relationship between whole and part. I cornered my critic with the crusher: It is literally impossible to deal with this complexity; you can only deal with parts on the basis of which you get better glimpses of what the whole is like. And the appropriate retort was: But how you actually approach and deal with the part must be influenced mightily by where you see it in relationship to the whole; that is, what you hope to do and the ways in which you go about it are consequences of how you think it is embedded in the larger picture.

What the years at the Psycho-Educational Clinic taught me was that the small voice should have shouted earlier in my stay there because as time went on I realized that if I had forced myself to confront what I did know about the community, and whom I knew in it, I definitely would have proceeded in different ways with different groups and different focuses. More important, such a confrontation would have told me what I did not know about the community, and whom I did not know, and how both types of ignorance would inevitably affect what I proposed to do. The fact is that I was using the term *community* without bothering to examine what its references were for me.

If I finally learned something, it is primarily because the clinic was created to deal with, among other important considerations, the myth of unlimited resources (Sarason, 1972). In his own way, George Albee (1954, 1968) had been yelling, with data no less, at the mental health movement to face up to the scandalous and socially irresponsible discrepancy between supply and demand. I was sympathetic to his message because I had come to see that what professionals characteristically do, with the best (or at least, not with the worst) of intentions, is to define a problem so that its solution requires *only* professionals, thus rendering the problem unsolvable (Sarason, 1971, 1972). As soon as you take this indisputable conclusion seriously, one of the questions you have to deal with is, How do I locate people who have the requisite skills but are not employing them, or who have the potential to acquire quickly some or all of the needed skills? How you think about this question (assuming your professional preciousness permits you seriously to pursue the question, if only for kicks) and the numbers you come up with will be determined by the scope of your concept of a community and the number of networks you can tap into. More correctly, the number of networks you can tap into is a criterion of the scope of your concept of a community. If you play with this way of thinking, you may find, as I did from experience, that the numbers you come up with are surprisingly large and that you are thinking about parts of the community ordinarily outside your interests and ken.

A concrete example follows. We were helping to create a new state facility for handicapped children (Sarason, Gorssman, & Zitnay, 1972). If you know anything about how such facilities are planned and created, you know why they become the graveyard for high hopes and for fantasies of innovative practice. The reasons are many, as I have pointed out elsewhere (Sarason, 1972), but high on that list is limited manpower. Our task was to locate people who had skills we needed and who would seriously consider giving them to us for free. We were not only looking for the volunteer who could answer the telephones or put stamps on envelopes or help in the kitchen; we also needed people with special knowledge and skills. Where were they and in what numbers? For the sake of brevity I shall start with the fact that we found ourselves in the office of the society editor of the local newspaper. We came away with a list of over 100 organizations, the degree of relatedness or overlapping among them, and some sound advice on how to go about our task. The important point in all this is that we learned a great deal about aspects of the community we never dreamed of as being either interesting or important for us. In practice, the scope of our networks was small, but potentially it was and did become vast, and our conception of the community broadened.

It could be argued that the concept of networks may be of some value for the purpose of understanding and broadening our conception of a community, and conceivably would be productive in dealing with the resource issue if one were so inclined. But was it not more than a little silly and wasteful to go the route we did rather than advertise? It would take me too far afield to justify (as I could) our approach in the specific case, but I wish to use the question to discuss the larger and crucial issue it raises: How does one get community support for what one is trying to do? How can one get support for what others in the community want to do and with which you are in sympathy?

My last three books (Sarason, 1971, 1972, 1974) have been concerned with the basis for and the processes of institutional and community change. In writing each of these books I had the unsettling problem of how many instances of failure and catastrophe I should describe of attempts by mental health professionals to implement their community orientation or programs. I say unsettling because I felt uneasy about being perceived as a cataloguer of unwitting disasters or as a dyspeptic observer of the current scene, especially because I did not feel that I was *that* much wiser than they. I do not think it was a wise decision to limit the number of cases because I have met a number of people who have reacted approvingly to what I have written but who go on to describe their activities in a way to suggest that my generalizations were not well comprehended. For example, one of the most frequent mistakes that is made is to neglect or vastly underestimate the importance of answering these questions: What individuals or groups will be directly affected by the proposed program? What issues of territoriality will it raise for which agencies, professions, and other interest groups? Who can be counted on to put obstacles in the way of the proposed program? Who has the power, actual or potential, to prematurely terminate the program? When you try systematically to answer these and related questions—and these questions refer to one's own organization as well as to external ones—you will find that what you propose to do impinges on networks radiating far into the community, that is, that what you propose to do will become related to quite an array of existing relationships. Indeed, performing this exercise is instructive in giving one a healthy appreciation of the myriads of interlocking networks that exist in a community. Unfortunately, an appreciation of this has always come *after* the program has failed, or has been aborted, or has fallen far short of the mark, or has been so transformed that its original goals are no longer in the picture. But even that is a too charitable assessment because in many instances the major "lesson" articulated is that there are a lot of stupid, selfish, power-hungry people in the community who feed on well-intentioned, health-giving professionals.

There is a problem in dealing with these questions that can easily be overlooked (it almost always is,) and once stated it is "obvious." Those who conceive the program, passionate and committed to a set of substantive ideas they consider innovative and needed, are not in the best psychological set to deal ahead of time with the radiating community consequences of their program. They are psychologically in a set in which optimism and hope and possession of their version of the truth obliterate a systematic approach to the question. In my experience, even when there is a sensitive awareness to these questions, one can predict that they will encounter in themselves two sources of resistance. The first is that it will take time, more time than they are willing or prepared to give. The second source is that they tap into existing networks to get soundings, they are likely to find— they will always find—nodes of opposition. They are, in fact, likely to find that their ideas can be expected to galvanize existing networks, near and far, in opposition to their program. Even if their proposal is to give away large sums of money to affected individuals or community agencies—to ask nothing of the community but to accept the money—they will encounter all sorts of opposition and criticism.

It is apparent, I hope, that in raising questions about consequences I have been leading up to the crucial point that a community venture requires support, the kind of support that one can count on to surmount the numerous obstacles that the answers to the questions indicated. And that is the point: The process of tapping into networks to obtain information and soundings is the first stage of the process of answering the question: How much support will we require from what networks to provide us with a fighting chance? And the chances are always fighting ones. It is beyond the scope of this article to pursue the processes of gaining support and the dilemmas of compromise.[2] I wish to conclude this part of my presentation by emphasizing that the root cause of the failures I have observed inheres in a conception of a community that ill prepared us for understanding its complexity and our actual and potential relationships to it, as well as for harnessing its resources behind our efforts.

What are the distinguishing characteristics of a community psychologist? In stating characteristics, I make no pretense at inclusiveness. He or she is a person who stands in awe of the discrepancy

---

[2] I will have little to say in this article about how community psychology has come to grips with issues of values, that is, how one justifies one's actions and programs in relation to community involvement. I have discussed this problem in some detail in Sarason (1974).

between first-hand experience of the community and the knowledge needed to comprehend its complexity. He or she is also a person who has made it a point to become familiar with that part of the social science literature that deals with the history and organization of communities, particularly as that literature bears on the ways in which communities are changing. It is this kind of knowledge that allows one to tolerate the discrepancy I described above because it provides a kind of compass to direct efforts to enlarge this first-hand experience. But the community psychologist is one who also knows that the picture of a community one gets from reading in the social sciences is painted in broad strokes and usually from a standpoint that does not in any direct way point to action for change. The community psychologist, precisely because he or she is involved in understanding *and* change, is one who learns that these broad strokes, while illuminating, are not sufficient for explaining myriads of interrelationships among networks in the community. It is like the situation of the clinician who knows from theory that the behavior and personality of members of a family are a function of various, specifiable factors in familial interactions, but who also has learned from practice how these factors can be differently manifested and patterned in different families. Community psychologists are pursuers of new knowledge and new networks in the community, not only because of immediate or long-term purposes but also because they see themselves as helping unrelated networks come into relationship with each other in light of their mutual needs. Community psychologists seek for themselves and others a sense of community (Sarason, 1974), and acceptance of this value requires them to play the "good-broker" role. They are not neutral about values, if for no other reason than that nobody is. But because they take on the label of *community* psychologist, they have come to grips with the shoulds and oughts of community functioning. Community psychologists lack the grandiosity which alone can permit one to believe that he (or his group) can change a community, but they possess the certainty that their efforts to understand and change a part of the community are doomed if in some way they do not conceptualize these efforts in terms of the larger picture.

Community psychologists are not clinical psychologists or mental health professionals. They are not superior to them, just different. They do not start with theories of the individual, and they are not absorbed by intrapsychic complexities. Pathological behavior may be of interest to them but primarily in the context of how resources are defined and used so as to maximize the psychological sense of community. They are wary of professional imperialism and preciousness because guildism, however well intentioned in its origins, resists community scrutiny and influence. Conflict is no stranger to them, but it is not the kind of conflict contained in traditional psychological theory in which the individual is usually figure and all else is ground. For the community psychologist, conflict stems from the different traditions, interests, and statuses and other characteristics of different groups, differences producing more or less impermeable boundaries among them—leading to a degree of ignorance of each other not explainable on or even very productively in purely psychological terms. The economics of the mind is one thing; the economics of a community are another. The politics of a family are important and fascinating but so are the politics of a community to a community psychologist. Sibling rivalry is a valid and productive construct for the clinician, but so is conflict among community groups for limited resources a stock-in-trade concept for community psychologists. The clinician seeks to utilize an individual's strength to combat his weaknesses; the community psychologist is not less sensitive to a community's strengths as weapons against its weaknesses. The clinician seeks allies, internal or external, to the individual. Building alliances is also second nature to the community psychologist.

The truth is that the community psychologist I have described does not exist, or hardly exists. Certainly, our training programs do not produce such a person. When World War II gave rise to modern clinical psychology, it was assumed—the way we assume that the sun will rise—that its viability required an alliance with psychiatry and the medical setting. For those of you who doubt this or were in elementary school at the time of the 1948 Boulder Conference, I suggest you read those proceedings. (I confess to some satisfaction in being part of a small minority at that conference who considered such an exclusive alliance as equivalent to aborting the potentialities of a differentiated and innovative social-clinical psychology.) As someone once said: It hasn't been all bad. I quite agree. Therefore, when I suggest that a viable community psychology needs allies I should not be interpreted as recommending other than a loose confederation among community psychology, ecological psychology, and the social sciences.[3] When modern clinical psychology was born, it had to con-

---

[3] I have elsewhere (Sarason, 1974) made the point that the characteristics of American social psychology—in its own ways an individualistic, experiment-worshipping fugitive from the social world in which we live our lives—provided no conceptual framework for either modern clinical psychology or the community mental health field. The absence of social psychology from the confederation is not an act of exclusion on my part but simply the belief that it has little to offer. Again, this is not intended as a way of manifesting any superiority on my part or that of the fields upon which I would base a community psychology. The fact is that when all of us entered the post–World War II era we were conceptually bankrupt before we began. Please remember that bankruptcy does not mean that one is without assets, just that one does not have enough assets to carry on one's business. I am petitioning for a reorganization.

tend with psychiatry, a professional war not yet over. (Why is it that, to my knowledge, there has been no doctoral dissertation on this professional fight? The ahistorical stance of clinical psychology and psychiatry is but one indication of why neither field could give birth to a productive community orientation.) Community psychology will not have to contend with such opposition. Indeed, my experience suggests that there are individuals in these allied fields who would be warmly supportive of attempts to forge new relationships. Note that I said individuals, not departments, because the modern university has many of the characteristics of a community, and the person who seeks to forge a new set of relationships to implement a new kind of program is faced with all of the issues I have already discussed. He or she has to use existing networks, tap into new ones, and develop a basis of support. Before we venture into the "real world" we have to solve the same problems in "our" real world, and from the standpoint of action and change the two worlds are similar. Before we save other people's worlds, we should first be able to demonstrate that we can save our own.

In concluding this article I would like to deal with a criticism directed at my position by a student. Paraphrasing his remarks:

> The way you describe community psychologists, they are remarkably similar to a lot of people in the community. Police, organized criminal syndicates, politicians, business people, fund raisers, and Mr. Joe Blow himself— all of them would say that what you are describing are persons with common sense who have lived in the real world and have tried to get something done. They will all tell you that you have to get to the right people, you have to learn who the right people are, and that you have to know the territory like the guy in "The Music Man" said. They would also agree with your criticism of professionals who screw things up when they want to do good in the community. What, they would say, do these professional do-gooders and bleeding hearts know about life in the real world? I would not be surprised if they looked on what you have said as another glimpse of the obvious described by another academic who does not know the difference between common and uncommon sense.

These remarks bothered me because there was a part of me that was ready to agree with my critic, and yet, if I agreed, if only in part, I felt that the strength of my position would be considerably weakened. Besides, even if I was convinced he was wrong, I was not convinced by my reply to him, and, of course, neither was he. Reflection, if not candor, forced me later to realize that what bothered me was the illness of professional preciousness. I wanted a community psychologist to be a distinctive and, perhaps, unique kind of person and, therefore, I was not going to look kindly at a criticism which said that far from being distinctive, the community psychologist was like a lot of other people. That thought forced me to go back and read Carl Becker's 1931 presidential address to the American Historical Association. The title of his address was "Every Man His Own Historian." In his paper—which I would make mandatory for anyone pretending to seek a liberal (liberating) education— Becker shows the communalities between Mr. Everyman (today it would be Mr. Everyperson) and the professional historian. I cannot present here Becker's arguments—they defy brief summary. But this quotation will give you the aroma if not the taste of the intellectual dish he serves:

> If the essence of history is the memory of things said and done, then it is obvious that every normal person, Mr. Everyman, knows some history. Of course we do what we can to conceal this invidious truth. Assuming a professional manner, we say that so and so knows no history, when we mean no more than that he failed to pass the examinations set for a higher degree; and simple-minded persons, undergraduates and others, taken in by academic classifications of knowledge, think they know no history because they have never taken a course in history in college, or have never read Gibbon's *Decline and Fall of the Roman Empire.* No doubt the academic convention has its uses, but it is one of the superficial accretions that must be stripped off if we would understand history reduced to its lowest terms. Mr. Everyman, as well as you and I, remembers things said and done, and must do so at every waking moment. (pp. 235-236)

Toward the end of his paper, Becker reassures the professional historian that he has both a common and an uncommon role to play:

> The historian, like Mr. Everyman, like the bards and storytellers of an earlier time, will be conditioned by the specious present in which alone he can be aware of his world. Being neither omniscient nor omnipresent, the historian is not the same person always and everywhere; and for him, as for Mr. Everyman, the form and significance of remembered events, like the extension and velocity of physical objects, will vary with the time and place of the observer. After fifty years we can clearly see that it was not history which spoke through Fustel, but Fustel who spoke through history. We see less clearly perhaps that the voice of Fustel was the voice, amplified and freed from static as one may say, of Mr. Everyman; what the admiring students applauded on that famous occasion was neither history nor Fustel, but a deftly colored pattern of selected events which Fustel fashioned, all the more skillfully for not being aware of doing so, in the service of Mr. Everyman's emotional needs—the emotional satisfaction, so essential to Frenchmen at that time, of perceiving that French institutions were not of German origin. And so it must always be. Played upon by all the diverse, unnoted influences of his own time, the his-

torian will elicit history out of documents by the same principle, how-ever more consciously and expertly applied, that Mr. Everyman employs to breed legends out of remembered episodes and oral tradition. (pp. 251-252)

"More consciously and expertly applied"—that is the kernel of the answer I wish I had given my student critic. We are similar to and different from Mr. Everyman and that should be a powerful reas-surance for the community psychologist. And if we forget that bond we have lost our roots and, as Becker says,"our proper function."

REFERENCES

Albee, G. *Mental health manpower trends.* New York: Basic Books, 1954.

Albee, G. W. Models, myths, and manpower. *Mental Hygiene*, 1968, 52, 168–180.

Barker, R. G. On the nature of the environment. *Journal of Social Issues*, 1963, 19(4), 17–38. (a)

Barker, R. G. *The stream of behavior.* New York: Appleton-Century-Crofts, 1963. (b)

Barker, R. G. *Ecological psychology. The stream of behavior.* Stanford, Calif.: Stanford University Press, 1968.

Barker, R. G., & Gump, P. V. *Big school, small school.* Stanford, Calif.: Stan-ford University Press, 1964.

Barker, R. G., & Schoggen, P. *Qualities of community life.* San Francisco, Calif.: Jossey-Bass, 1973.

Barker, R. G., & Wright, H. F. *One boy's day.* New York: Harper & Row, 1951.

Becker, C. Every man his own historian. In *Essays on history and politics.* New York: Crofts, 1935.

Gladwin, T., & Sarason, S. B. *Truk: Man in paradise.* New York: Wenner-Gren Foundation for Anthropological Research, 1953.

Kelly, J. G. Book review of R. G. Barker & P. Schoggen's *Qualities of community life. Community Psychology*, 1975, 20, 193–195.

Price, R. H. The taxonomic classification of behaviors and situations and the problem of behavior-environment congruence. *Human Relations*, 1974, 27, 567–585.

Price, R. H. & Blashfield, R. K. Explorations in the taxonomy of behavior set-tings: Analysis of dimensions and classifications of settings. *American Jour-nal of Community Psychology*, 1975, 20, 335–351.

Sarason, S. B. *The culture of the school and the problem of change.* Boston, Mass.: Allyn & Bacon, 1971.

Sarason, S. B. *The creation of settings and the future societies.* San Francisco, Calif.: Jossey-Bass, 1972.

Sarason, S. B. *The psychological sense of community. Prospects for a community psychology.* San Francisco, Calif.: Jossey-Bass, 1974.

Sarason, S. B., Grossman, F. K., & Zitnay, G. *The creation of a community setting.* Syracuse, N.Y.: Syracuse University Press, 1972.

Commentary to
Chapter 12

*Beginning with my first professional job, at the Southbury Training
School, I have worked in or around schools. As will become clearer
in the last paper in this collection, I always believed that psychology
in general and clinical psychology in particular should be an intimate
part of the educational scene if they wanted to maximize their contributions to public welfare. Very few psychologists shared that belief,
which is why, when clinical psychology became a significant part of
American psychology after World War II, it allied itself with the
medical-psychiatric setting. It never made sense then, and events over
the past three decades have confirmed my prediction that the potentialities of clinical psychology for the public welfare would be trag-
ically restricted if it became embroiled in the culture of American
medicine. One could argue that clinical psychology was as unsophisticated about the culture of schools as it was of medical-psychiatric
settings. This may be true, but whereas clinical psychology was always a second- or third-class citizen in medical-psychiatric settings, it
had always enjoyed incomparably higher respect in the schools. In
addition, the possibilities for prevention of problems were incomparably greater in schools than in medical-psychiatric settings.*

*For a short period in the 1960s, diverse kinds of psychologists
became very interested in schools, particularly from the standpoint
of changing curricula, racial-ethnic attitudes, organizational structures,
and relationships with communities. For a brief moment it seemed
that psychologists understood what might be gained if psychology
were to make a major commitment to the public schools. It was a
very brief moment, however, because it became evident that psychologists did not understand the culture of schools or the nature of
institutional change, and they did not know that the major features
of today's schools could not be comprehended without knowledge of
the traditions and social history of the society. If psychologists lacked
these understandings, it was largely because psychological theories
were focused on individual organisms for whom society, culture, and
social history were a globbish background. A psychology of individual
minds is no basis for understanding, let alone changing, long-standing
social institutions. During the 1960s I respected and even applauded
the efforts of psychologists to change schools so that they would be*

more intellectually stimulating and interpersonally rewarding for everyone in them. I continued to respect the purposes of these psychologists, but my applause turned to boos when I observed repeatedly how their ignorance of the school culture forced them into self-defeating behavior. These observations, together with the near-total immersion of the Yale Psycho-Educational Clinic in school settings, led me to write The Culture of the School and the Problem of Change *(1971). As I write these words in late 1980, that book has been through fifteen printings. The sales of the book to psychologists have been minuscule, and I shall run the risk of appearing arrogant by saying that those sales figures say far more negative things about the substance and directions of American social psychology than about the quality of the book. Social psychology is social in the sense that it is riveted on individuals and interactions among them—the attitudes they bring with them and the ways those attitudes change as a consequence of those interactions. It is social in the sense of having an interpersonal or small-group focus. It is not social in the sense of placing these interactions in the context of a highly differentiated society that has a distinctive culture and ideology, reflected in and reinforced by governmental, political, educational, religious, and financial systems of institutions.*

Although this article is dated after the previous one, it was written first. The two articles, very different on the surface, have common themes. The first theme is how hard but crucial it is to put into words the assumptions that have been so successfully implanted in us by our socialization into the society; most people live their lives unaware of the sources that determine what they will consider "right, natural, and proper." The second theme is that the unverbalized nature of these assumptions has two frequent consequences: the assumptions restrict the universe of alternatives available to us for explanation or action, and they are potent obstacles to institutional change. In this article I use the teaching of reading in the early grades to illustrate these points—and no one will deny that the attempts to prevent reading failures, or to remedy reading problems, have met with very little success. Why has the reading problem proved so intractable? It is precisely when a problem has been intractable to efforts to overcome it that we must learn to search for those unverbalized assumptions without which our actions make no sense but with which we head for trouble.

12

A "Cultural" Limitation of System Approaches to Educational Reform

This paper points out a limitation on the knowledge that the public educational system is intimately related to or interlocks with other systems, e.g., political, economic, class, professional. This knowledge was, until relatively recently, not recognized on the public policy level which heretofore reflected the fiction that schools were a kind of social oasis protected from the rest of society, presumably to insure that the education of the young would not be corrupted by the evils of society. It was a myth nourished by rhetoric and the processes of denial of social realities. The myth was forever exploded by the events of the past two decades. The public educational system was and always has been tied to, affected by, or related to all other major social systems. The recognition of these intersystem relationships gave rise to two tasks: to understand these relationships better (more realistically), and to devise means by which they could be harmoniously interlocked toward the goal of improving education. One has to be thankful that these intersystems realities have been uncovered because they have given a rise to a good deal of theorizing and actions providing a base for critical scrutiny. It is, I assume, an advance when realities supplant myths, even though the process is inevitably painful and turbulent. If I aim to emphasize a limitation of systems thinking and practice, it is in no way to deny their fruitfulness. To illustrate the major point of this paper, I shall look at the actual uses of the new knowledge in terms of their impact on a major education problem: the failure of many children to read even near their grade level.

S. B. Sarason, "A 'Cultural' Limitation of System Approaches to Educational Reform," *American Journal of Community Psychology* 5, no. 3 (1977): 277-287. Reprinted with permission of Plenum Publishing Corporation.

There are many school children who cannot read at or near their age-grade level. Another glimpse of the obvious is that this situation has been intractable to efforts at remediation. One can always find teachers in our "worst" urban schools whose pupils do learn to read, but even when their approach and methods are adopted by other teachers the results are disappointing. It is probably fair to say that any policy based on the assumption that the overall problem will be licked either by certain kinds of teachers or methods has failed or will fail. I do not regard this conclusion as pessimistic, if by that is meant either that I believe that many children do not have the capacity to read or that there are no alternatives to policies that say that if more money was spent, teachers better trained and motivated, and more interesting materials employed, the printed word would come to have glamor for nonreading pupils. What I am pessimistic about is the capacity of educational policy makers to confront the reality of their failures and to entertain alternative ways of thinking. This difficulty is not peculiar to educational policy makers. It is a difficulty we all share for the simple reason that culture (any culture) inevitably provides us with ways of thinking and unexamined values that constrict the universe of alternatives for action we can think about (Sarason, 1971; 1974). Unless we understand and act upon this point— consciously to make the effort to transcend the limits our culture imposes on us—we are not likely to meet social crisis and challenge in effective ways. If I illustrate this point in the context of systems thinking and practice, it is because this context, so relatively new and potentially productive, allows me to discuss the more basic issue of culture, thinking, and action. I am less interested in discussing a limitation of systems thinking and practices than in the mixed blessings of culture.

There are some who say that our educational system has failed, reading being only one of its failure symptoms. But what do people mean by the "educational system"? From one standpoint it might be said that many people have come to see that the educational system is far more complex than they ever imagined—or, more accurately, that it has become more complex than ever before. The educational system is not a collection of buildings staffed be diverse and hierarchically organized professionals, administered by a central office staff, all of whom are responsible to a public board who in turn are instrumentalities of state government. It is now known, as it could have been earlier, that the public educational system was intimately related to colleges and universities, that the system was always related to the community and its political system, that religion (the constitution notwithstanding) was an influential force, and that economic values and resources were always at or near center stage. And with the beginning of federal intervention the system became even more complex. In short, to describe and understand a single school or school system requires that we deal with other systems or agencies the actions of which make some kind of an impact on the educational system. (Note that I have not mentioned the law enforcement and public welfare systems which, formally and informally, have much commerce with the educational system.)

What has been gained by recognizing a complexity in which everything is related to everything else? Judging from the myriads of efforts to change the educational system, the question has been answered in several ways. One radical answer, precisely because it purports to get at the root of the matter, is that we are dealing with a new multiplicity of power relationships from which will emerge new alignments supplanting the previous sources of policy and power. The teacher union movement, growing ever stronger and seeking collective-bargaining rights for ever enlarging geographical areas, seems intent on influencing the educational system in other than narrow "bread and butter" matters, e.g., the More Effective School program proposed by Albert Shanker. Far less cohesive, militant, or programmatic is the community control or community participation movement, a large urban area phenomenon in which different racial and ethnic groups are dominant. Both movements seek a redistribution of power as a way of rescuing a failing educational system. Both maintain that if they succeed, the quality of children's educational experience will change in ways that make for productive learning, e.g., more children will really learn how to read. And both movements seem to be setting the stage for a head-on collision.

The rationale for the government-sponsored Project Open (Bigelow, 1971) is based on the clear recognition of the many systems with which the educational system interrelates, and on the assumption that one can develop a strategy or process by which they can share power at the same time that power struggles among them can be diluted or even avoided, i.e., mayors, legislators, school personnel, and community leaders can educate each other about their need for mutual help in improving the educational system. Like the teacher union and community-control movements, Project Open recognizes the existence of power conflicts, but unlike them it does not seek to produce a "winner." Project Open is not a substantive program but a process which hopes to keep interrelated systems "open" to each other. On the national scene, Project Open is of no significance and I mention it here because it is so clearly a response to the knowledge that the educational system interrelates with other social systems with which it must deal more directly and openly than ever before. Differences aside, Project Open, like the other responses to the need to redistribute power to formulate and implement educational policy, shares the belief that if it is successful it will ultimately and desirably improve the quality of the educational experience. None of these responses say explicitly that they will "solve" the reading problem, but it is implicit in all of them that they are to be judged not by whether they win or lose in terms of power (shared or not) but by the degree to which they transform the educational experience of children who are now doomed to be "failures."

There have been other responses to the knowledge of the complex interrelationships between the educational and other systems, but they are difficult to categorize. It would be only somewhat of a distortion to say that they have faced the knowledge and decided not to deal with it. Take Head Start, for example, which rested on the diagnosis that ghetto schools were inhospitable learning environments, that they were insensitive to community needs and changes, and that their teaching personnel were culturally or racially different than pupils and parents. Another part of the diagnosis was that the deplorable schools were a reflection of neglect by the community's political and economic power structures. In the days of the war-on-poverty programs there was a kind of national *mea culpa*, a national self-indictment that left no major institution uncriticized. Head Start did not deal with these larger issues but proceeded as if it could inoculate preschoolers against the diseases they would encounter when they entered the public schools. The implicit diagnosis upon which Head Start rested was far more sophisticated than the strategy which emerged. Alternative schools are also examples of avoiding "the systems" by deliberately trying to be as independent of them as possible.

The most radical of all responses are those which seek literally to supplant the existing educational system by one which permits parents, by some kind of voucher system, to determine where they want their children educated, i.e., educational facilities would be in a "competitive market," and their survival would largely be a function of their quality (Flygare, 1973). The need to compete for the parental dollar would, presumably, eliminate educationally submarginal and marginal people and facilities. If a school was not helping its children to learn, for example, it would not be in business very long. On the surface, at least, the voucher proposals seem to be directed against the perceived defects and failures of the educational system in its narrow sense. But when one even cursorily examines their likely consequences, it seems clear that they aim "to free" schooling not only from the existing educational establishment (local, state, and federal) but also from its dependent and debilitating relationships with the political and economic systems. The teacher unions, of course, have to be utterly opposed to such proposals if only because they obviously threaten their capacity to use all of these systems to gain their goals. The growth of teacher unions was, in part, due to their recognition and use of the fact that the educational system was integrally related to, and ultimately controlled by, other social systems. Any effort to separate the educational system from other systems is a threat to union strength. I do not say this critically but only to illustrate the point that teacher unions and proponents of voucher proposals seem to share identical assessments of the interrelationships among the different systems, although they use this knowledge to come to diametrically opposed conclusions.

All that I have said are glimpses of the obvious. It is obvious, however, only because the events of the last two decades have, so to speak, hit us over the head with the result that we see interrelationships we did not see before—at least most people did not see or could not acknowledge before. Of course we knew before then about interlocking social systems, and that the educational system mirrored the characteristics of the larger society. But few knew it with that sense of detail and immediacy that informs action and planning. Most of us wanted or were taught to believe that what went on (or could go on) in schools primarily reflected intrasystem forces. We looked on our schools as naively as people used to look at professional sports. We did not want to believe that both were activities highly interrelated with economics, politics, race, religion, and social structure.

On a purely descriptive level what has been gained by the recognition of the complex interrelationships between the educational and other systems are different ways of changing the educational experience to prevent or dilute the consequence of pupil failure. It should be noted (and emphasized) that none of these ways spells out why it will have desirable effects on the educational experience of children. For example, it is mystifying why any of these proposals will decrease the number of children who cannot read or read at a level far below their grade level. In each instance the assumption seems to be that by changing inter- and intrasystem characteristics, predictably desirable changes will occur in the educational experience of children. Such an expectation is a hope not justified by an explication of why these system changes should have these outcomes. For example, economists have a sufficient understanding of our economic system to be able to say that when that system is altered by changes in fiscal or monetary policies, certain groups or parts of the economic system will likely be affected in certain ways. And we also know that changing the economic system already reflects, and will subsequently reflect again, the working of the political system; and in the past two decades we have learned that changes in the interrelationships between the economic and political systems always have consequences for the educational system. In short, we know a fair amount about how intra- and intersystem changes will differentially affect people. This kind of knowledge is precisely what is lacking when extrapolations are made from actions to alter the intra- and intersystem characteristics of education to what will happen to children, e.g., those who cannot read. I am not maintaining that these actions will have no desirable effects on adults in or out of the system. Indeed, it is my impression from my experience as well as those described by others that these efforts have had liberating effects on different groups of adults: teachers, parents, administrators, public officials, etc. But I have been most unimpressed by the effects on children's educational experiences. This failure, I suggest, is a cultural phenomenon in the sense that we are all, in different degrees, unwitting prisoners of what our culture teaches us about what schools are and should be, so that it is inordinately difficult for us to conceive of another way in which realities may be ordered. This was beautifully demonstrated to me in a seminar I was conducting for city school administrators. Not surprisingly, I was sounding off in one-track fashion on the theme "That the more things change the more they remain the same."[1] In the course of discussion, one of the participants said in a somewhat puzzled and despairing manner: "Every now and then after I have visited a school I play the following game. I ask myself to remove myself from my training and job and to come up with a new and better way in which schools might be organized and function. I am not the only educator who plays this game, and frequently when we get together in a group we gravitate to some version of the game. Why is it that what we come up with shows such startling similarities to what schools *are*?" What his comments indicated was a dawning awareness that culture was both ally and adversary; ally because it gives order and meaning to our lives, and adversary because it does its job so well we cannot conceive of a different order. It requires a major crisis and up-

---

[1] This is the central theme of my book *The culture of the school and the problem of change* (1971). The present paper derives from that book which contains several examples of how difficult it is for those within or related to a particular kind of setting to become conscious of how their "picture" of the setting is based on unexamined, cultural givens. This difficulty, restricting as it does the "universe of alternatives" we allow ourselves to consider, is discussed at greater length in my book *The creation of settings and the future societies* (1972). My most recent book *The psychological sense of community. Prospects for a community psychology* (1974) further pursues the issue of how culture restricts consideration of the relations between values and action.

heaval, usually over a sustained period of time, before new values and ideas can be seriously considered.

No one would argue against the proposition that any social system reflects the culture. In agreeing to this proposition, however, few realize that one of the effects of culture is that it provides us with a picture of reality that seems "natural" and precisely because we learn to see it as natural we are unable to question it, e.g., to conceive of another way of organizing the world. If, for example, you are brought up in a culture that "says" you *should* eat three meals a day, you unreflectively regard it as not only natural but right. Culture not only shapes our perceptions but our values as well. It is likely, therefore— indeed it is very likely—that when we seek to change that reality, we leave untouched or unexamined the cultural givens that are the underpinnings of our perceptions and actions. Concretely, when we attempt to change the educational system in its intra- or intersystemic aspects, we run the risk that we are leaving unexamined the cultural givens. Let me illustrate this with the problem of reading failures in our urban schools.

There have been scores of proposals to prevent or reduce the frequency of reading problems. None of them makes any sense in the absence of one implicit assumption: young children (e.g., between 5 to 8 years of age) *should* learn to read. Anyone who has any doubt about the force of this assumption should visit any first- or second-grade classroom (or kindergarten for that matter) in any urban school. To almost all people the validity of the assumption is obvious. What are these early grades for if not to learn to read (and to learn numbers and computation)? Hasn't it been the traditional function of these early school experiences to establish the basis for reading competence? It may be that our past practices are no longer adequate, that our curricula are outmoded and unstimulating, that our classes are too big, that our teachers need a different professional preparation, that we have not spent enough money, that our educational theories are wrong and incomplete, that we need more basic research. Granted, some would say, that any or all of these are correct, how can one suggest, as I do, that young children should not have to learn to read at any specific time? Is that not further victimizing the victim? The disbelief and emotion that my position elicits is testimony that a treasured but unquestioned picture of reality is being challenged, that a cultural given is being criticized. It is not unlike the response that initially greeted the ideas of social security, unemployment insurance, abortion, easy divorce, the legalization of marijuana, and equality for women—or the idea that two parallel lines will meet in space. In each of these instances people's conception and perception of how the world is and should be organized were challenged and their response was predictable. *I am not suggesting, of course, that any challenge of a cultural given is valid either in terms of values or practical consequences.* I am only emphasizing how inordinately difficult it is for us to recognize how much of our outlook is culturally overlearned, literally to an unthinking degree. But the suggestion that young children should not have to learn to read is not offered only for illustrative purposes. It goes, I think, to the heart of the matter because it raises possibilities far more healthy than we now have. After all, there are millions of children who, for all practical purposes, will be non-readers, and there is no reason to believe that we are on the road to remedying the situation.

Several arguments help people to overcome their initial incredulity to the idea that young children should not have to learn to read. (When on formal occasions I have pursued the matter, I start with the suggestion that a law be passed making it illegal to teach young children unless there is good evidence that they are begging to be taught.) The first is that I am not opposed to children learning to read. Second, I am dead serious in suggesting that the idea be applied to all young children, not only ghetto children. Third, there is no reason to believe that our schools will collapse and our society will deteriorate further or faster. Fourth, there is reason to believe that many children who now are not reading in the early grades will wish and learn to read later. Fifth, and this is most applicable to the many elementary school personnel with whom I have talked (and argued), they can generate no basis for optimism that what they are now doing or what others are proposing that they do will have a discernibly desirable or general effect. Sixth, it is not a new idea: John Dewey said much the same thing decades ago, and acted on it successfully in developing his school at the University of Chicago. Seventh, teaching children who are either not ready or motivated to read frequently aggravates rather than helps the problem. (This last point is somewhat similar to Wendell Johnson's concept of the "diagnosogenesis" of stuttering: the child does not begin to stutter until after the parents have made their diagnosis. It is a variant of the self-fulfilling prophecy.)

When people (by no means all) overcome their initial incredulity, at least to the point where they recognize that the world will not come to an end if young children are not required to read, I have come to expect a second manifestation of what happens when a cultural given is challenged. *What will we do with the children?* This, understandably, is verbalized most clearly by teachers. "If we are not permitted formally to teach reading, what *do* we do? Do we become babysitters? Entertainers? Storytellers? Television specialists? Whatever it is we become, we are no longer teachers. Of what use is our professional training?" What is being reflected, of course, are conceptions of role, structure, and learning which are not only interrelated but accepted and reinforced by our schools, universities, and the larger society. They are conceptions so successfully ingrained in us that we are rendered impotent to act when they are rendered inoperative. For example, a decade ago I conducted a weekly seminar for beginning elementary school teachers in the New Haven school system. They were a bright, highly motivated, liberal arts educated group who had chosen to work in inner-city schools. We met each Wednesday. One of the meetings was Wednesday after the assassination and funeral of President Kennedy. There was no school on Monday (the funeral) and, if I remember correctly, school was also cancelled for Tuesday. When I came into the seminar room there was much talk about two things: the teachers' reactions to those troubled days and, more important for our purposes, the difficulty they had "teaching" the children who wanted only to talk about the assassination. Several teachers stated explicitly that the children had learned "nothing" that day, and others expressed their guilt about having taken time to discuss the children's questions about and reactions to the assassination. When teachers are prevented by events from following a predetermined curriculum which by its very nature defines specific goals, pacing, and the structure of teacher-children relationships, they do not regard themselves as teachers, and children learn "nothing." If teachers feel that way it is because they, like the rest of us, are reflecting what the culture "says." They reflect the culture; they are not reflective about it. The most unfair mistake we can make (and it has been made many times) is to scapegoat teachers, as if we do not share with them the same cultural givens about what a teacher and formal schooling are and should be.

"*What will we do with the children?*" In that question is wrapped up some of the most important differences between school and non-school perceptions of learning, differences deliberately sought and fostered by the culture. There is never a doubt in anyone's mind (children, teachers, parents) that there is (and should be) a discontinuity between learning in and out of school. For many children that discontinuity is catastrophic, as it is for teachers who seeing the children as inadequate or unready or unsocialized, redouble their effort to sharpen the discontinuity. Rist (1973) has recently provided a detailed description of this process based on his participant observations of a kindergarten class which he followed for 3 years. He is quite critical of teachers, the school system, and teacher-training programs which he views as manifestations of our society's exploitive and discriminatory economic, social class, and racial structure. At no point does Rist raise the possibility that the tragedy he describes so well, in part may stem from the basic assumption he shares with teachers: young children should learn to read. Rist gives no indication that if he transformed teachers, classrooms, and school systems (indeed, all of society) according to his values, he would tamper with the basic academic objectives of the early grades. He would select teachers differently, change their preparation, humanize teacher-child relationships, and make the boundaries between school and community more permeable. But the basic objectives of schooling in the early grades would remain as they now are, presumably because the changes he would bring about would create the conditions in which these children would learn. I am suggesting that his unreflective acceptance of these traditional objectives would set severe limits to what would be accomplished; his acceptance of objectives puts him in the position of reinforcing society's acceptance and, I may add, that of our teacher-training centers. Put in another way: unreflectively accepting that young children should learn to read requires accepting and reinforcing certain aspects of the schools' intra- and intersystemic aspects.[2]

It is apparent, I hope, that a limitation of a systems approach to reforming education is that it is not intrinsically rooted in or directed towards a critical examination of assumptions, values, or objectives which our culture makes seem "natural." For certain objectives of reform I assume that this limitation is not serious, although intuitively I think this is never the case. For objectives which have to do with reforming life in the classroom, this limitation is always present and serious, if not fatal. We may redistribute power within and between systems, we may bring about more open discussion and effective cooperation among those who are waiting, we may infuse the educational system with more money and personnel—we may do all of these things and yet not markedly effect the major educational problems which initially regalvanized the reform movement. I would maintain that we are and will continue to be disappointed with our efforts because we are prisoners of cultural givens about schooling that are now counterproductive. These cultural givens have made for a self-defeating discontinuity between formal and informal learning.

---

[2]There are practical problems with my suggestion that young children should not have to learn to read. For example, high mobility of urban populations means high pupil turnover, as any inner-city teacher well knows. Consequently, my suggestion would have to be implemented in a system. Please note that at present this very high rate of pupil turnover, interacting with the structure and objectives of the early grades, has adverse effects on children. This is not the place to go into the problems with my suggestion. Suffice it to say that I am a firm believer in Murray Levine's maxim of "problem creation through problem solution."

This degree of discontinuity has been discussed in a recent paper by Scribner and Cole (1973). It is a paper based on cross-cultural experiences and studies, and deserves the closest reading. Let us listen to the implications they draw from an analysis of cognitive consequences of formal and informal schooling in cultures quite different than our own.

> We have maintained that the problems and techniques of the school are not the problems and techniques of practical life or the traditional home. The school's knowledge base, value system, and dominant learning situations and the functional learning systems to which they give rise are all in conflict with those of the student's traditional culture. If we take this opposition seriously, certain implications follow for the educational policy.
>
> For one thing, it is not necessary to look further for explanation of the difficulties formal education may present to people who rely heavily on informal education as their basic method. The problem does not lie "in them." Searches for specific "incapacities" and "deficiences" are socially mischievous detours.
>
> Second, if many of the demands of formal schooling are by their very nature discontinuous with those of everyday life, it seems unreasonable to expect masses of children to cope successfully with them so long as they perceive the school to be a hostile institution. Yet this is exactly the situation in many poor and minority neighborhoods in the United States and in many third-world countries. The antagonism the schools generate by their disrespect for the indigenous culture and by ignorance of its customs almost guarantees the production of nonlearners. *While indigenous control of the schools cannot by itself undo the basic opposition between informal and school-based education, it is surely a necessary precondition for their reconciliation.*

The sentences I have italicized seem to be making one of the major points I have tried to make: intra- and intersystemic efforts at educational reform are necessary, but unless they are realistically tied to an understanding of the present discontinuities between formal and informal schooling, they will end up by proving that the more things change the more they remain the same (Sarason, 1971).

A final comment has to do with two recent publications. The first is *Youth: transition to adulthood*, a report of the Panel on Youth of the President's Science Advisory Committee (1973). The second is: *Scholarship in society, a report on emerging roles and responsibilities of graduate education in America* (Educational Testing Service, 1973). What is noteworthy about these reports, which concern suggested changes in formal schooling from junior high through the graduate school levels, is the clear recognition that discontinuities which

Scribner and Cole (1973) discuss must be drastically weakened. As I read these different reports it struck me as ironic that at all levels of formal schooling analogues of the question "why should young people be required to learn to read" are being asked. The irony resides in the fact that at each level of formal schooling questions are being asked that are genotypically identical to those being asked at all other levels, but there is little indication that the identity is perceived as broadly as it should. I suppose we should not expect that those recommending important changes in graduate education should perceive their conceptual kinship with those whose focus is on the high school or the elementary school. However, I am tempted to be mildly encouraged by the fact that at all these levels the cultural givens, the heretofore unreflectively accepted "shoulds and oughts," are being questioned. It is only on the basis of such reexaminations of what has been "natural" and traditional that we will have the basis for deciding what we want intra- and intersystemic change to accomplish.

REFERENCES

Bigelow, D. (Ed.). *The liberal arts and teacher education.* Lincoln: University of Nebraska Press, 1971.

Flygare, T. J. An abbreviated voucher primer. *Inequality in Education*, 1973, No. 15, 53–56.

Rist, R. C. *The urban school: A factory for failure.* Cambridge, Mass.: MIT Press, 1973.

Sarason, S. B. *The culture of the school and the problem of change.* Boston: Allyn & Bacon, 1971.

Sarason, S. B. *The creation of settings and the future societies.* San Francisco: Jossey-Bass, 1972.

Sarason, S. B. *The psychological sense of community. Prospects for a community psychology.* San Francisco: Jossey-Bass, 1974.

Scholarship in society, a report on emerging roles and responsibilities of graduate education in America. Princeton, N.J.: Educational Testing Service, 1973.

Scribner, S., & Cole, M. Cognitive consequences of formal and informal education. *Science*, 1973, 182, 553–559.

Youth: transition to adulthood. Report of the Panel on Youth of the President's Science Advisory Committee, June 1973.

Commentary to
Chapter 13

World War II plunged psychology into the public arena as never be-
fore. With each succeeding postwar year, the institutions of psy-
chology became increasingly related to and involved in matters of
public policy, directly and indirectly, and therefore in social action.
The theme was onward and upward, but—as I indicated earlier—not
from my standpoint. The 1960s and their aftermath were a debacle
for psychology and for the social sciences generally. In previous articles
I had discussed certain features of American psychology that con-
tributed to the debacle, such as scientism, the limitations of an in-
dividual psychology, an at-best superficial understanding of the nature
of our society, and an ahistorical stance. One other feature I had been
mulling over for years had to do with theories of and research in prob-
lem solving. My first stab at ordering my thinking was in a paper I pre-
pared for the Nebraska Symposium on Motivation in 1961, entitled
"The Contents of Human Problem Solving." It was the expectation
of those who invited me that I would be talking about anxiety, but
I had already had my fill of anxiety research, and so I used the occasion
to raise some questions:

Interest in and research about the problem-solving process requires no
defense. I do feel, however, that it is legitimate and necessary to ask why
the bulk of studies in this area have focused far more on the processes than
on the contents of human problem solving. In my opening sentence I indicated that in studies of problem solving the subject is *presented* with a
problem and the way in which he solves it is observed and inferred. I emphasize the word "presented" in order to distinguish this approach from
one which focuses on problems which can be said to arise spontaneously in
the course of human development. For example, and I shall have more to
say about this later, I assume that all children in all cultures at some point
arrive at the problem (without the problem necessarily presented to them
by another person) of how to explain anatomical differences between the
sexes. What are the different ways in which children experience the
problem? What is the relation between the contents of this problem and
those of concurrent problems? How does the content of this problem
change over time? How are the different solutions (without necessarily
understanding the process of solution) related to the solution of other
problems? What environmental factors affect the contents of the problem?

Here again I was being critical of the prepotent tendency to focus on problem solving in formal testing situations and to neglect naturally occurring problem-solving situations. Implicit in the case material on which I based my discussion was the idea that the problems in these naturally occurring tasks were not "solved" in a once-and-for-all fashion; that is, they would undergo transformations that required resolution of the problem. That idea was implicit, however, and I did not see that I was using the term solving *in the natural science sense; that is, once you solved the problem you did not have to solve it again. Clinically, I knew that the contents of these problems were never solved in a once-and-for-all fashion. Problem-solving research in psychology dealt only with problems that had solutions in the natural science sense of solution. The Nebraska paper coincided with the beginning of the Yale Psycho-Educational Clinic and my total immersion in social action. Those days there was a surfeit of "solutions" for the myriad social problems that had forced their way onto the public agenda. I found myself increasingly uncomfortable at the ease with which people came up with solutions and at the belief, expressed* ad nauseum, *that, if we had a better scientific understanding of the problems, they would then, and only then, be amenable to real and lasting solutions. What I came to see was that the traditional conception of solution was inappropriate for social action. It was not only inappropriate, it was harmful, disillusioning, misleading, and self- and socially defeating. Why that was so and how it came about are discussed in the article that follows.*

13

The Nature of Problem Solving in Social Action

You cannot understand a past era unless it leaves some kind of record of evidence of what people said or did. We look back from a vantage point that allows us to scan for myriad evidence, a scanning impossible for anyone in that past era. We like to believe that our vantage point is high enough, our vision unclouded by all of those factors that put blinders on those who lived in that past era, and that we have the accrued knowledge, skill, and wisdom to explain not only what happened, or how forces were related to each other, but also the why of it all. And the why of it all almost always has to do with ways of thinking that give order and direction to daily living. What lends fascination to historical constructions and reconstructions is in the process of deducing or intuiting what people in that era took for granted. But if the process is fascinating, it is inherently problematic. For one thing, there are many vantage points; so many, in fact, that it is literally impossible for one person or group to climb them all. No less serious for those who have to believe that they are on the road to truth, and that the road has an end, is that reconstructions of the past always reflect what we from our present vantage points take for granted. Can you deduce what people in a far off era took for granted without what you take for granted affecting your conclusions in ways that you cannot know but people in future eras will think they know? The process of historical reconstruction inevitably says as much about the present as it does the past. If history strikes so many people as uninteresting and irrelevant, it is, in part, because they do not understand that what we call history is literally manufac-

S. B. Sarason, "The Nature of Problem Solving in Social Action," *American Psychologist* 33, no. 4 (April 1978): 370–380. Copyright 1978 by the American Psychological Association. Reprinted by permission.

tured by the present. When Henry Ford, that self-made sage, said "history is bunk" he was saying a good deal about himself and many others in our society, far more than he was saying about the past. That was obviously less true, but still true, in the case of Gibbon's *Decline and Fall of the Roman Empire*.

The social-historical stance has not been a dominant feature of American psychology. An amusing but illuminating example. Back in the later forties the American Psychological Association began to accredit graduate programs in clinical psychology. An APA committee came for a site visit, and part of their time was spent talking with our graduate students. At the end of the visit I talked with one of the committee members who expressed satisfaction with our program, with one exception. He had asked one of our graduate students if he had read Köhler's *The Mentality of Apes*, and the reply was: "No one reads that any more. That's old hat." We both laughed, very uneasily. Both of us were pre–World War II trained psychologists and very much aware that as a result of the war the face of psychology was being changed. For both of us, the Henry Ford type of statement by the graduate student presaged something disquietingly new in psychology, but it was hard to put into words. The downgrading of the historical stance was not new, but if what this student said was at all representative of his generation of psychologists, the small place of history in psychology would shrink to near extinction. If I had to say what bothered me, it would be that I placed a lot of weight in living on the sense of continuity, a belief not created or particularly reinforced by my training in psychology. Beyond that personal need my unease had little conceptual substance. But something told me that what the student said was very important and I have been trying ever since to make sense of it. The first conclusion I came to was that there was really nothing new in what the student said. By virtue (among other things) of psychology's divorce from philosophy and marriage to science, history in psychology became a lot of narrow histories depending on the particular problem that interested you. That is to say, if you were interested in reaction time to a type of stimulus, you had the obligation to know what others in the past had done and found. This obligation served several purposes: to deepen your knowledge of the particular problem to avoid repeating what others had done, and to increase the chances that what you were going to do would shed new light on the problem. This might be called the rational justification of the use of history. But, as is always the case, there were non-rational factors at work. In fact, justifying the use of history only on rational grounds, or describing it as a completely rational process, should have been warning enough that these justifications were incomplete and misleading. Behind these justifications were some beliefs and hopes. One of them was that you were going to add something new to an understanding of the problem precisely because you were building on knowledge provided by others from the past.

In the scientific tradition knowledge is cumulative: you either add a new brick to the edifice of knowledge so that it looks different or, better yet, you destroy the edifice and present your colleagues with a foundation for a new and better structure. One part of this tradition says that knowledge is cumulative, the other part says that your contribution is proportionate to how much past knowledge you have rendered obsolete. You use history, so to speak, with the hope of destroying its usefulness. This kind of attitude or hope is subtly but potently absorbed by young people entering scientific fields, and I believe it has been particularly strong in psychology, less because of psychology's youth as a scientific endeavor and more because of its self-conscious desire to identify with that endeavor. This has tended to produce still another belief: if a study was done ten years ago, it is unlikely that you will learn much from it; if it was done twenty years ago, the chances are even smaller; and if it was done before World War II, don't forget it but be prepared quickly to do so. Put in another way, it would go like this: "we have come a long, long way in a relatively short period of time and there is not that much from the past that is usable to us now. What is more worrisome than whether we are overlooking anything from the past is whether someone in the present is rendering what I am doing as wrong or obsolete." Köhler studied apes during World War I. Obviously, the odds are small that he has anything to say that is important to the here and now of psychology! Yes, he probably belongs in the Museum of Greats but you only go to museums when you are not working. My purpose is neither to discuss nor question the implicit and explicit uses of history in scientific research. What I wish to suggest is that these uses (and, therefore, perceptions and conceptions of the past) have been very influential in shaping people's attitudes toward the significances of history in general. That is to say, among all those who think of themselves as scientists there has been a noticeable tendency to view the social world as having been born a few days ago. This should not be surprising when one considers the status and functions society has given to science. Within the confines of its own traditions science long has been on an onward-upward trajectory in the course of which it has displayed a seemingly boundless capacity to solve its problems. This did not go unnoticed by society as it saw that in solving its problems science could also contribute to the welfare of society. Scientists and the public came to agree that the deliberately impractical goals of science (knowledge for knowledge's sake) had very practical implications. No one ever said it, and perhaps no one ever thought it, but the agreement between science and society contained a "message": society had problems *now* and science could be helpful in solving them *now* or *in the foreseeable future*. There was no disposition to recognize that the relatively ahistorical stance of science might be mischievously inappropriate to social problems. Put in another way: the pride that science took in rendering past scientific knowledge obsolete; the view of its past as more interesting than it was usable; its concentration on now and the future—these stances fatefully determined the degree to which, and the ways in which, society's problems would be placed in an historical context. This type of influence seemed proper and productive as long as the findings of science had two types of consequences: one was of the technological, thing-building or thing-creating variety, and the other was of the illness prevention or the illness curative variety. It may be more correct to say that the nature of the influence went unnoticed as long as there was near universal social acceptance of what science seemed to be able to do. As long as society posed essentially non-historical questions for science, science came up smelling technological roses. Agriculture, industry, medicine, the military—they asked the kinds of here and now questions to which the findings of science could be applied.

It is hard to overestimate how total identification with science eroded whatever significance social history had for psychology. For one thing, it seriously limited the capacity of the field to examine its past to illuminate its present, i.e., to try to fathom how its view of the past (and its projections into the future) may be a function of the myth making present. For another thing, it blinded psychology to the obvious fact that any field of human endeavor is shaped by forces beyond its boundaries, and that its structure and contents can never be wholly explained by that endeavor's narrow history. For example, can one understand the history of behaviorism or psychoanalysis by restricting one's self to what behaviorists and psychoanalysts did and said? Boring did his best to sensitize psychologists to "zeitgeist" but his efforts have been honored far more in the breach than in the practice. "The spirit of the times" is such an apt metaphor because it warns us that what we think and do, what we think we are, what we say the world will be—all of these in part reflect influences that are time-bound and hard to recognize. The word "spirit" (an uncongenial one in psychology), like the concept of the unconscious, reminds us that as individuals or fields we are affected by forces near and far, known and unknown, inside and outside.

At its best, social history serves the purpose of reminding us that we, like those of past eras, are very biased, time-bound organisms. We differ in all kinds of ways from those of past eras but one thing we clearly have in common: we breathe the spirit of our times. If we use social history for the same purpose we do a table of random numbers, we stand a little better chance of avoiding the worst features of un-controlled bias. At the very least, sensitivity to social history makes it hard to ignore several things. First, despite all the diversity among human societies, past and present, each dealt with three problems: how to dilute the individual's sense of aloneness in the world, how to engender and maintain a sense of community, and how to justify living even though one will die. Second, each society defines and copes differently with these problems and, as a society changes, as it inevitably does, the nature of the definitions and copings changes. Third, these changes, more often than not, are not recognized until people see a difference between past and present definitions and copings. Fourth, the three problems are always here and there in the life of the individual and the society, but not in the sense that inani-mate matter is here and there. Fifth, these are not problems that people have created, and they can never be eliminated or ignored. Sixth, any planned effort to effect a social change (as in the case of scientists who seek to apply their knowledge and skills for purposes of social change) that does not recognize and understand the history and the dynamics of these three problems will likely exacerbate rather than dilute the force of these problems.

Applying scientific and technological knowledge and skills in social action is not like applying paint on a wall, except as both appli-cations literally obscure what you may not like to look at. Scientists who enter the world of social action like to think of themselves as possessed of the basic knowledge and problem-solving skills of their science, and they often have a feeling of virtue because they are apply-ing these to practical social issues. What they fail to see is that because science does not start with the three problems, that science in no explicit way recognizes or is controlled by them, science *qua* science has no special expertise to deal with them. Everyone knows the old joke about the graduate student who had learned about latin square design and was looking for a problem that fitted it. There is a way of looking at science and seeing some similarity with the student. Science has learned a lot about problem-solving, but when it looks beyond its confines to the arena of social problems, it has tended not to ask what are the "basic" problems there but rather to seek problems that fit its problem-solving style: clear problems that have unambiguously correct solutions. The separation of science from disciplines concerned with social history will always obscure from science that not all basic problems in nature can be molded to its problem-solving models.

SCIENCE AND SOLUTIONS

Before World War II academic psychology never quite made up its mind whether it was a social or biological science. The image of the laboratory was very attractive. After all, look at what had been discovered in laboratories, and wasn't society grateful? If psychology was to earn society's gratitude, and also be accepted by the older sciences, you needed, among other things, a certain kind of place where problems could be analyzed, dissected, studied. A laboratory was a place where you solved problems. You could study problems outside of a laboratory but that meant that you had drastically reduced the chances of finding solutions to basic problems. In a laboratory you could manipulate variables, and, obviously, you could not arrive at rigorous solutions without experimental manipulation of variables. The image of the laboratory contained several features: physical isolation, clearly stated problems, experimentation, hard work, solutions. It was such an attractive image that few psychologists seriously questioned its appropriateness for their new field. There were psychologists for whom the laboratory was not an appropriate place to study problems but they did not question the other features of the image. Their task, they would say, is the same but harder because experimental manipulation outside the laboratory was so difficult. They felt inferior, and were made to feel inferior, because it was so unlikely they could "really" solve any problem. The "real" general laws of human behavior were going to be found by studies done in certain ways and places. Science could not tolerate sloppiness of method and uncertainty of solution.

Take, for example, pre–World War II psychology's view of psychotherapy. My guess is that psychologists would not have been in favor of making the practice of psychotherapy illegal. They would have agreed that if people had personal problems there should be trained individuals to try to help them. But, they would have added, psychotherapy is an art, and a pretty poor one at that, and do not confuse it with science or technology derived from science. So, they could have been asked, what are *you* doing about it? The answer would have been that psychological science is seeking the basic laws of human behavior and not until the basic questions are clarified, studied, and solved in the most rigorous ways can a foundation be provided for truly effective psychotherapeutic practice. It's like building bridges: basic science had to solve a lot of basic problems before engineers could build bigger and better bridges. It is, they said, going to take us time, and one of the worst things we could do would be to start studying an applied problem like psychotherapy to the neglect of more basic psychological issues. Let us not kill the goose that lays the golden eggs, as an eminent psychologist once said.

Now, if you knew something about social history, and you had the courage, you could have asked: "is it possible that these problems are of a human and social nature that are not solvable by science? Is it not obvious that in the chasm between your scientific findings and solutions, on the one hand, and the realm of human affairs, on the other hand, is a mine field of values for the traversing of which your science provides no guide? If we can build magnificent bridges, or develop life extending vaccines, is it only because of basic problem-solving research or is it also because society wanted those fruit from the tree of science? Just as technology depends on basic science, don't both depend on or reflect the wishes of the larger society? What will happen if and when the social world changes and the relation between society and psychology is altered so that psychology is asked and willingly attempts to solve social problems it never encountered, and never could encounter, either in the laboratory or through employment of any of its research strategies? Will psychology be found inherently wanting?

These were questions that could not be raised in psychology before World War II. Some of these questions were explicitly raised by one psychologist, J. F. Brown in his 1936, *Psychology and the Social Order*, but no one paid him much mind. In the midst of a social catastrophe, the Great Depression, Brown saw the crisis in psychology and this he was able to do because social history in its Marxist version had become part of his conceptual framework. His was not a parochial mind, witness his attempt to bring together Marx, Lewin, and Freud. Lynd, a sociologist, raised similar questions in his 1939 book, *Knowledge for What?* Having studied Middletown before and after the Great Depression, Lynd, like Brown, questioned the traditional directions of the social sciences and asserted their conceptual and moral bankruptcy.

In one crucial respect Brown and Lynd were in basic agreement with an underlying assumption of a science: all problems of society, like those in the rest of nature, had solutions. The problems may be of a different order, and the ways of studying and controlling them may require new theories and methodologies, and their solutions may be a long way off, but they were solvable. Who would deny that the creativity and ingenuity that had unravelled the mysteries of the atom, exemplified in the work of Rutherford and Bohr, or that allowed Einstein to supersede Newton, would falter when faced with the problems of social living? But what if these problems were not solvable in the sense to which science was accustomed?

The concept of solution in science is by no means a clear one and it is beyond my purposes to examine the different and overlapping meanings that concept has been given. In one respect, however, the lay and scientific understanding of a solution is very similar: a problem has been "solved" when it does not have to be solved again because the operations that lead to the solution can be demonstrated to be independent of who performs them, and when the solution is *an* answer to a question or set of related questions, and there is no longer any doubt that the answer is the correct one. If there are competing answers, the problem has not yet been solved. So, when geneticists around the world were trying to "solve" the genetic code, they could agree on only one thing: someone would find *the* answer. And the answer would be of the order of "four divided by two is two." There is or will be only one correct solution. There are times, of course, when the solution about which there is consensus is proved wrong and then everybody is off and running to find the "really" correct solution. The correct solution always raises new questions but at least the earlier question does not have to be solved again. The question was asked, the solution was found, and now for the next question.

Problem-solving is a venerable and sprawling field in psychology. I wish to note two of its characteristics. The first is that almost without exception the human subject is presented with a problem that is solvable, although the correct answer may be arrived at in different ways. Indeed, how an individual arrives at a correct solution has been considered no less important than the fact that he got a right solution. One of the major influences of the Gestaltists (Wertheimer, Koffka, Köhler, Lewin) on research in problem-solving was in their emphasis on the psychological factors and processes (e.g., set, insight, perceptual reorganization) that preceded solution. The graduate student's opinion notwithstanding, Köhler's (1925) studies of problem-solving in apes is still instructive reading, as is Wertheimer's (1959) classic *Productive Thinking*. The fact remains, however, that the distinctive emphasis of the Gestaltists had meaning in the context of solvable problems. It is not fortuitous that Wertheimer illustrates his ideas by a description of how Einstein solved problems with which physicists of the time had been grappling.

A second characteristic of the problem-solving literature is that the types of problems used in research almost defy categorization. It is an exaggeration to say that each researcher develops his own stimulus problem but it is not a gross exaggeration. It would be understandable if someone concluded that when researchers used the words "problem-solving," they were far more interested in "solving" than they were in "problems."

Let me illustrate the significance of these two characteristics of the problem-solving literature by asking this question: why, for all practical purposes, is there nothing in this literature on how artists solve their problems? For example, what was the problem or problems Cézanne was trying to solve? This question has nothing to do with his personality, although it does with his times. What was the cognitive substance of the problem, how was he trying to solve it in a visual form, what made for such a long struggle, and did he solve the problem? Several answers could be given to the question. One would be that we cannot be sure what the problem was, and even if he were alive we could not accept his version of the problem. How do you justify studying problems whose clarity and formulation you know ahead of time must be of dubious status, and there are no known ways of determining what the "real" problem is? If you are fuzzy about the nature of the problem how can you ever state criteria by which to judge successful outcomes? And what do we do if Cézanne said: "In this painting I solved the problem, in that one I did not." Do we accept his judgments, and what have we learned by doing that? And what do we learn from fellow artists who are awed by Cézanne's accomplishments? Their judgments permit no firm conclusions about the relationship between problem and solution. Besides, not every artist, then or now, agrees either about the substance of Cézanne's artistic problems or artistic solutions. A final answer might be: Cézanne is a great artist but his problem-solving accomplishments cannot be understood and judged in the way the works of great scientists can be. In short, they would say Freud was right: before the artist you throw up your hands. These are problems that are not science's cup of tea. There is problem-solving that does not fit the researcher's requirements of a clear, manipulable problem and unambiguous criteria for the correct solution. So, science has always left that problem alone, albeit from a stance of superiority. The problems of social living were also left alone until the emergence of the social sciences, led by economics. Just as the natural sciences had developed laws about the non-human world, the social sciences would seek the laws of human society, not only for the purposes of explaining the workings of society but for controlling it. They would be the embodiment of Plato's philosopher-kings. Apparently they were not impressed with the fact that Plato saw the problems of social living as so difficult to understand and cope with, requiring of philosopher-kings such a fantastic depth of learning and wisdom, that one could not entrust social responsibility to them until they were well along in years. And to my knowledge, Socrates infrequently answered a question and never solved a problem. He was too impressed with man's capacity for self-justification and self-deceit. Neither Plato nor Socrates ever assumed that the accomplishments of Greek scientists reflected a model of problem asking and problem-solving that was appropriate to the development of the good society. In the millenia that followed there were many people who took a similar position. Science never really came to grips with them, least of all social science.

SOCIAL ACTION

Let us now turn to a moment in history when the workings of impractical science led to a most practical product, one that our scientists and society desperately wanted. It was a moment that at the same time that it illustrated the fruitfulness of scientific problem-solving exposed its inappropriateness for solving social problems. I refer, of course, to the successful solution of all the problems, theoretical and technical, leading to the harnessing of atomic energy for military purposes. As soon as it became evident that a successful atom bomb was in the offing, some scientists began to ask themselves questions: to use it, how to use it, and how the seemingly endless uses of atomic energy for human welfare could be exploited? They saw a problem, many problems, and as in the case of Cézanne, the substance of the problem was by no means clear. The end result of a successful solution seemed clear: a world in which the destructive uses of atomic energy was rendered impossible or nearly so, and its uses for human welfare maximized. But how do you go from here to there? What was the bearing of the scientific tradition on that problem?

As best as I can determine none of the scientists thought they were dealing with a scientific problem. They recognized they had been catapulted into a social world that was fantastically complicated, constantly changing, and seemingly uncontrollable. It was not even a maze because that image conjures up entry points, stable pathways, and some kind of end point. The social world was not a maze. It was not even a cloud chamber because that is a device rationally constructed to record and measure predictable events. It may be a world of facts and events but it was ruled by passions. It is ironic in the extreme that at the same time that the world saw these scientists as at

the apogee of human achievement, they saw themselves as angry, be-
wildered, impotent people. They became like most other people: passionate, committed, partisan, rhetorical, and irrational. Those are not
characteristics foreign to scientific controversy and investigation, but
the morality of science and the critical eyes of the scientific community are effective controls against the undue influence of these
characteristics. If you suspect a fellow scientist of lying and cheating,
or of just being a damn fool, you have ways of finding out and spread-
ing the word. But that means there is consensus about the rules of
the game. The social world was not the scientific world. As a physicist
friend once said to me: "What the hell kind of world is it?" He used
exactly the same tone of petulance-anger that Professor Henry Higgins
uses in *My Fair Lady* when he asks why can't women be like men?
My friend also went on to say (paraphrased), "I can't deal with a
world where everybody has his own definition of the problem, facts
are an intrusive annoyance and of tertiary importance, where who
you are is more important than what you know, and where the need
to act is more decisive than feeling secure about what the consequences
will be." And he concluded with this: "I will stick to my world where
there are answers, and if I don't find them someone else will." When
the atomic scientists entered the world of social action, that world
could not be molded to fit their accustomed problem-solving strategies.

But, many social scientists thought, those were atomic scientists
and one should not be surprised that when they left the world of
minute matter and entered the world of human matters, they faltered.
After all, they were not social scientists whose stock in trade was
human matters. The fact is that up until World War II the social sciences had contributed to our understanding of the social world, but
with one noteworthy exception these contributions were mainly descriptive, or analytic, or historical. They were not contributions stemming from the social scientist's effort to participate in and solve social
problems. Like the natural scientist, the social scientist was the dispassionate observer, and deliberately so, who sought to formulate
clear questions to which clear answers could be obtained. He saw his
task as understanding the social world, not changing it. The one exception was economics which for decades had an intimate tie with the
practical world of government, business, industry, and finance. Early
on, economists not only described the world as they saw it but they
drew conclusions about what should or should not be done. They
were listened to, and they took responsible positions in the social
arena. Heilbronner (1961) has aptly called them the "worldly philosophers." They lived, so to speak, in two worlds: the scientific problem-
solving world, and the world of social action.

It was the Great Depression that really made the world of social action accessible to increasing numbers of economists. The underlying assumption, of course, was that economists had knowledge and skills that could inform public policy and action. If during the thirties the atomic scientists had developed firm friendships with their university colleagues in economics (unlikely events in the community of scholars), they would have learned much earlier than they did that scientific knowledge as power in the social arena is one of a different order than it is in the research community; that in the social arena one is always dealing with competing statements of a problem and there is no time or intention to experiment in implementation with one or another of the formulations; that the choice of formulation has less to do with the traditions, value, world outlooks, and the spirit of the times; that the goal of social action is not once-and-for-all solutions in the scientific sense but to stir the waters of change, hoping and sometimes praying that more good than harm will follow; that the very process of formulating a problem, setting goals, and starting to act not only begins to change *your* perception of problems, goals, and actions but, no less fateful, the perceptions of *others* related to or affected by the process in some way. *In the phenomenology of social action, problem changing rather than problem-solving is figure, and you know what that does to solutions regardless of how you define them!*

World War II opened up many opportunities for social scientists to be in social action or policy related roles. That was truly the first global war bringing us into contact with scores of different cultures and peoples. So, as never before, anthropologists became socially important people. And sociologists and psychologists were even in short supply. World War II forever changed the social sciences. They were exposed to new problems, and much that they thought they knew was proved either irrelevant or wrong. More important, they tasted the heady wine of influence and action and they liked it. Government needs us, they said, and government seemed to agree. At least one noted psychologist (Doob, 1947) had his doubts and his brief paper beautifully describes the naive scientist in the world of social action. Doob's paper is noteworthy in two other respects. First, his recognition that in social action the scientist *qua* scientist is like a fish out of water: dead. " . . . where social science data are adequate or where social science itself can provide only principles or a way of approach to a problem, the social scientist must hurl himself into the debate, participate on an equal or unequal footing with men and women who are not social scientists, toss some of his scientific scruples to the winds, and fight for what seems to him to be valid or even good. A strict adherence to the scientific *credo* in such circumstances leaves the social scientist impotent and sterile as far as policy is concerned." Second, the fact that Doob early on learned that if he responded seriously to his and others' need for mutuality and community, even if some of those others were opponents, social action could be rewarding despite the fact that one never knew whether one was having an intended programmatic effect, i.e., that one was solving a problem.

In the aftermath of World War II the government became both patron and employer of social science. After all, the argument ran, if the government respected and supported social science research, as it did research in the biological and natural sciences, the social atom might be split and its energies harnessed for the greatest good of the greatest number. For twenty years after World War II the social sciences became, and with a vengeance, vigorous, quantitative, theoretical, and entrepreneurial. If you wanted to solve in a basic and once-and-for-all way the puzzles of individual and social behavior, you needed resources of the wall-to-wall variety. True, it would take time to learn to ask the right questions, to develop the appropriate methodologies, before you can come up with the right answers. What we are after are those bedrock laws of social behavior and process that will allow a society "really" rationally to diagnose and solve its problems. Give us time (and money) and you will not regret it. In the meantime if you think we can be helpful to you with your current problems, please call on us. And call they did, and go they went. The results have been discouraging and shattering, discouraging because of the lack of intended outcomes, and shattering because it calls into question the appropriateness of the scientific-rational model of problem definition and solution in social action. Nelson (1977), a noted economist, has summed it up well in his recent book, *The Moon and the Ghetto.* (I am sorry he did not retain the original subtitle: A study of the current malaise of rational analysis of social problems. The malaise is real and, to my knowledge, Nelson is one of the few who has dared to articulate what others only think about.)

The search for "the Great Society" entailed highly publicized efforts at turning the policy steering wheel. Broad new mandates were articulated— the war on poverty—and specific policies were designed to deal with various aspects of the problem. The histories of these departures clearly identify the key roles often played by research reports, social science theory, formal analytical procedures. More recent years have seen an increasing flow of proposals for organizational reform: vouchers for schools, health maintenance organizations, greater independence for the post office, a national corporation to run the passenger railroads, pollution fees, revenue sharing.

It is easy to trace the intellectual roots of many of these ideas. The techno-science orientation has come later, and never has had the thrust of the others. Nonetheless the intellectual rhetoric has been strong, and has generated at least token efforts to launch the aerospace companies on problems of garbage collection, education and crime control, and programs with evocative titles like "Research Applied to National Needs."

The last several years have seen a sharp decline in faith, within the scientific community as well as outside, regarding our ability to solve our problems through scientific and rational means. Those who want to get on with solving the problems obviously are upset about the loss of momentum. It is apparent that many of the more optimistic believers in the power of rational analysis overestimated that power. There are strong interests blocking certain kinds of changes. Certain problems are innately intractable or at least very hard. But the proposition here is that a good portion of the reason why rational analysis of social problems hasn't gotten us very far lies in the nature of the analyses that have been done. John Maynard Keynes expressed the faith, and the arrogance, of the social scientist when he said, "The ideas of economists and political philosophers, both when they are right and when they are wrong, are more powerful than is commonly understood. . . . I am sure that the power of vested interests is vastly exaggerated compared with the gradual encroachment of ideas." But surely Abe Lincoln was right when he made his remark about not being able to fool all of the people all of the time . . .

In addition to their clumsy treatment of value and knowledge (a problem that seems to infect analysts generally), analysts within each of the traditions have had a tendency to combine tunnel vision with intellectual imperialism . . . Members of the different traditions have had a tendency to be lulled by their imperialistic rhetoric. This has often led them to provide interpretations and prescriptions that the public, and the political apparatus, rightly have scoffed at. Failure to recognize the limitations of one's own perspective has made analysis of problems that require an integration of various perspectives very difficult. Indeed a kind of internecine warfare obtains among the traditions over the turf that lies between them.

Nelson illustrates his position using day care, breeder reactor programs, and the SST.

Nelson argues that there are inherent limitations to the scientific problem-solving model as the basis for social action, and he also suggests that these are problems that are inherently intractable. The very word "intractable" is foreign to the scientific tradition. In science, problems may be extraordinarily difficult but they can ever be viewed as intractable, and if some fool says a problem is intractable it is because he is not posing the problem correctly or he does not have the brain power to work through to the solution. In science, fools are people who say problems are intractable. In the realm of social action, fools are people who say all problems are tractable.

THE CHALLENGE OF INTRACTABILITY

Why is it so difficult for people, particularly scientists to entertain, let alone accept, the possibility that many problems in social living are intractable, not solvable in the once-and-for-all-you-don't-have-to-solve-it-again fashion. I have already given one part of the answer: science has been such a success in solving so many of the problems in nature that people became persuaded that the dilemmas and puzzles of the human social world would likewise become explicable and controllable. In fact, people in Western society were so persuaded that it became an article of unquestioned faith. And when religion's hold on people's minds began to disappear and the scientific outlook and enterprise took its place, it tended to go unnoticed that one article of faith (the world is divinely ordered) had been supplanted by another (the world, animate and inanimate, is ordered, knowable, and controllable). And the tendency of science to be ahistorical in general, particularly in regard to social history, effectively obscured for people that the rise of modern science not only coincided with the Age of Enlightenment but was its major beneficiary. And few things characterized that age as did the belief in the perfectibility of man and society. As Becker (1932) so well described, the heavenly city of St. Augustine would be built on earth, not through divine inspiration but through man's reason. Science could not recognize the possibility of intractable problems, and like the religions it supplanted it purported to give clear direction and meaning to living.

What would happen if one accepted intractability, which is no less than to accept the imperfectibility of man and his society? What would keep us going? How would we justify our individual strivings and our commitment to social action? What happens to the idea of progress? What will permit us to look forward to tomorrow? Do we seek, as some people do, new religious experiences that tell us we are not alone in this vast world, that there are solutions to the problems of living, and that mortality can open the door to immortality? And that last question, I submit, contains the substance of the real challenge of intractability to science in that it says that man needs to deal with three facts: he is inevitably alone with himself, he needs others, and he will die. These are facts that create problems but they are not the kinds of problems that fit into science's problem-solving model. Leaving religion aside (although it is true for many believers), the problems created by these facts need to be solved again, and again, and again. At different times in our lives the same problem has a different answer.

It has not gone unnoticed that the wonders of science and technology have had little or no effect on society's capacity to help its members feel less alone in the world, to enjoy a sense of community, and to help them cope with anxiety about death. Some would argue that the failure of science to start with and to be governed by these facts of human existence has exacerbated the pain associated with them. And when value free science entered the realm of human affairs, it exposed its naivete, its ignorance of social history, its hubris, and its blindness to man's need to deal with his aloneness, to feel part of and needed by a larger group, and to recognize and not deny his mortality. This is what the atomic scientists learned, or should have learned.

There is a malaise in all the sciences. For the first time in modern science, as well as in modern western society, people are questioning whether the fact that science and technology can accomplish a particular feat is reason enough to do it. In psychology we have been brought up short by the fact that as adherents to science we do not have license to conduct research in any way we wanted. We are accountable and that means that we should feel and nurture the bonds of similarity and communality between ourselves and the people we study. It is the difference between *knowing* that you are studying people, like yourself, and not "subjects". Society does not exist for the purposes of scientists. It is arrogance in the extreme to look at society from a noblesse oblige stance, expecting that the gifts you give to it will be responded to with gratitude, not questions or hesitations. Today, both among scientists and the public, there is the attitude that one should look a gift horse in the mouth.

What bearing does this have on social action? So let us talk about Norway. As you know, several years ago they found a lot of oil under the Norwegian sea. Far from this being greeted with hosannas and visions of a bountiful future, Norwegian leaders reacted with a kind of fear. What could happen to their society if they plunged into the development of the oil fields and began to collect the billions of dollars from the sale of oil? What would be the consequences for Norwegian culture, for their sense of continuity with their past, for their sense of community? A decision was made to go as slowly as possible, to give priority to what they regarded as the important issue in living! The Norwegians know that they live in a world they cannot control, that they will be subject to pressures within and without their society to develop the oil fields quickly and fully, that they may be unable to act in ways consistent with their needs and values. They may not be able to have it their way. Indeed, we can assume they will fall short of their mark. What will keep them going is what is wrapped in what a poet said: "Life takes its final meaning in chosen death." That may sound melodramatic but only to those who cannot understand that the fact of death informs the experience of living. We live each day as if we are immortal, although our rationality tells us how silly a basis for living that is. If our own rationality does not tell us, we can count on all sorts of events and experiences to shock us, not into the recognition of the fact that we will die, but into confronting how we justify why we have lived and how we planned to live (Becker, 1973; Sarason, 1977). And when scientists confront those questions, and each one does at one time or another, they frequently find that there was a lot they took for granted they wish they had not. But that is the fate of everyone. At each vantage point in our lives we see our history differently.

As for the scientist who enters the arena of social action (and that may be in different roles), he would do well to be guided by the values he attaches to the facts of living in much the same way that the amazing Norwegians are trying to do. That will present him with a type of problem (and transform his concept of solution) to which his scientific models are inappropriate and may even be interfering. He will find himself dealing in persuasion, not only facts; the problems will change before and within him; he will not be concerned with replicability because that will be impossible; there will be no final solutions, only a constantly upsetting imbalance between values and action; the internal conflict will not be in the form of "Do I have the right answer?" but rather of "Am I being consistent with what I believe?"; satisfaction will come not from colleagues' consensus that your procedures, facts, and conclusions are independent of your feelings and values, but from your own conviction that you tried to be true to your values; you will fight to win not in order to establish the superiority of your procedures or the validity of your scientific facts, concepts, and theories but because you want to live with yourself and others in certain ways.

Most scientists who entered the arena of social action have left it bloodied, disillusioned and cynical. They came with data and solutions, but even when they had neither they assumed that their training and capacity for rational thinking, their ability to pose clear problems and find appropriate methods leading to solutions, would establish their credibility as well as their right to an important role in rational social change. Most of them did not realize, if only for their lack of knowledge or respect for social history, that they were fully agreeing with Karl Marx who had said that it was not enough to try to understand the world. You had to change it and in a scientific way! Marx considered himself a scientist and the arrogance of scientism permeated his writings and actions. He had his theory, he stated the problems, collected his data, developed procedures, and had no doubt about the correct solution. And what scorn he had for his unscientific opponents! But Marx did not fool himself about what was behind his science, indeed prior to it. He saw man pathetically alone, separated from others, afraid of living and dying. Unfortunately, his dependence on his science led him to give priority to methods dictated by that science, and not by what those methods meant *at that time* to man's plight. The solution to that plight was put off to the distant future. In the meantime, trust Marx's scientific theory and procedures. Look what it explained and promised!

The scientist is committed to seeking and saying his truths and he must not be concerned with whose ox is being gored, an imperative science has never questioned because to do so would be to destroy the enterprise at its foundation which is, of course, moral in the sense of describing how scientists should live with each other. To the extent they live together on the basis of that imperative, scientific problems can be solved. In the social arena, whose ox is being gored cannot be ignored. It can, of course, be ignored, but history contains countless examples of how bloody the consequences can be. And yet, there are times when one takes a position and acts, knowing that the oxes of other individuals and groups will be gored. But somewhere along the way one should be aware that as important as the desire to prevail over your opponents is the need on both sides to feel some bond of mutuality. Winning no less than losing can increase one's sense of loneliness and decrease the sense of belonging. In science, how you did something is no less important than what you say you found. Some would say that how is more important. There are hows in social action, but of a very different cast, so different that it becomes understandable why so many scientists who entered the arena of social action faltered. They could not unlearn fast enough to start learning that the nature of problem-solving in the kitchen of social action bore no resemblance to what they had been accustomed. It is not a kitchen for everyone. But as my favorite president liked to say: "If it's too hot in the kitchen, get the hell out".

Even if you can get out, you will still be dealing with the same issues in your personal life and social circle. But even as a scientist, a new problem has arisen. I refer, of course, to the growing sentiment, already reflected in certain legislation, that what science studies, and the ways it conducts its studies, will be determined by the larger society. And one of the diverse factors behind that determination is the feeling that despite man's dazzling capacity to gain new knowledge and skills, to open new vistas for human experience, perhaps even to create new forms of life, he still feels alone, socially unconnected, unhappy in living and fearful of dying. It is a very hot kitchen, not one that the wonders of science and technology have been or will be able to air-condition.

What I have said is no excuse for inaction or pessimism, or any other attitude that only deepens the sense of aloneness, or accentuates the lack of community, or makes facing the end an intolerable burden. Nor have I in any way intended to denigrate science or intellectual endeavor. There is a difference between science and scientism, between modesty and arrogance, between recognizing limitations and seeing the whole world from one perspective.

Social action takes on a very different quality when it is based on or controlled by certain facts and values. In a recent book some colleagues and I (Sarason, Carroll, Maton, Cohen & Lorentz, 1977) describe an effort over a three and a half year period to develop and sustain a barter economy network of relationships the purposes of which were to deal more effectively with the fact that resources are always limited and people have a need for a sense of community. I should emphasize that it was an effort not only to increase people's access to needed resources but to do it in a way that also widened and deepened their sense of belonging. The members of this network range from high school students to researchers from different colleges and universities. It is an ever expanding network of human relationships that makes it a little easier, and sometimes a lot easier, to cope with personal and intellectual needs. Central to the story we tell is a remarkable woman we call Mrs. Dewar whose distinctive characteristic is the ability to scan her world to see and create opportunities whereby people unknown to each other are brought together because each has something the other person needs. There is resource but no money exchange, and people stay together and have call on each other.

The problem-solving literature is not helpful in trying to understand a Mrs. Dewar or several others like her we describe. None of these individuals has dealt with solvable problems defined in the traditional scientific sense, but they have transformed their worlds. How they did it is no less important than why they did it, but their distinctiveness in social action lies in the way they put the whys and hows together. In these days when social scientists, suffering from the burnt child reaction, are either retreating from the world of social action or scaling down their claims to credibility, they would be well advised to pay attention to people like Mrs. Dewar who are not burdened by the concept of "problems" but whose thinking and actions are explicitly powered by the concepts of "opportunities" and "matching," concepts in the service of a clear vision of what makes learning and living worthwhile.

REFERENCES

Becker, C. L. *The heavenly city of the eighteenth century philosophers*. New Haven, Conn.: Yale University Press, 1932.

Becker, E. *The denial of death*. New York: Free Press (Macmillan), 1973.

Brown, S. F. *Psychology and the social order*. New York: McGraw-Hill, 1936.

Doob, L. W. The utilization of social scientists in the overseas branch of the office of war information. *American Political Science Review, XLI* (No. 4), 1947, 649–677.

Heilbronner, R. L. *The worldly philosophers*. New York: Simon and Schuster, 1961 (paperback).

Köhler, W. *The mentality of apes*. New York: Harcourt, Brace & Co., 1925.

Lynd, R. S. *Knowledge for what? The place of social science in American culture*. Princeton, N.J.: Princeton University Press, 1939.

Nelson, R. *The moon and the ghetto*. New York: W. W. Norton, 1977.

Sarason, S. B. *Work, aging, and social change. Professionals and the one life-one career imperative*. New York: Free Press (Macmillan), 1977.

Sarason, S. B., Carrol, C., Maton, K., Cohen, S., & Lorentz, E. *Human services and resource networks*. San Francisco: Jossey-Bass, 1977.

Wertheimer, M. *Productive thinking*. New York: Harper, 1959 (Enlarged edition).

Commentary to
Chapter 14

In this, as in several of the previous papers, I direct attention to the fact that American psychology has been a psychology of the individual organism. In the previous papers I tried to show how limiting that kind of psychology is for understanding and dealing with the larger social world, whereas in this paper I suggest that it is no less limiting in the conduct of our individual lives. The emphasis here on our individual lives derives from the fact that I had just finished writing Work, Aging, and Social Change *(1977,1) which was based on interviews with individuals, young and old, in the professions. In conducting the interviews with new or would-be professionals, I was struck by how poorly they understood the micro and macro social structures within and about which they were making crucial life decisions. It was not that I expected these young people to be sophisticated social scientists and was disappointed that they were not, but rather that I was taken aback by the degree of their ignorance of how contexts were shaping their thinking and of how the characteristics of the contexts they sought to become part of might shape their lives. I could say they were naive and self-centered, but I would be subject to the very criticisms I was voicing if I thought I was explaining very much by these individual characteristics.*

In conducting interviews with older professionals, I was struck by their poignant awareness that their youthful stance and expectations had ill prepared them for what lay ahead: how the structure, boundaries, traditions, and ambience of the organizations in or with which they worked—the world "out there"—had forced important alterations in their internal worlds. As one of these people put it: "When I was young I thought the world was my oyster but in fact I was the oyster well shielded from the surrounding world." What was there about our society and its educational constitutions that made it so likely that young people would vastly underestimate the infiltrating power of external forces and vastly overestimate the role of internal forces in their lives? It was a question that psychology could neither address nor illuminate, precisely because it was almost exclusively an individual psychology.

Why had American psychology gone in this direction? Had it always had this emphasis in the modern era? In pondering these ques-

tions as I was writing this paper, I concluded that I had a great deal to read and think through; a few years later that conclusion lead me to write Psychology Misdirected: The Psychologist in the Social Order *(1981, 1).*

14

Individual Psychology: An Obstacle to Comprehending Adulthood

One of the most obvious features of our society is that it is not organized for the individual. Over the span of life each of us encounters obstacles, choice points, and phenomenologically new problems that are stressful and potentially defeating of our hopes. This may be true of any society, past and present, but a case can be made that today the points of conflict between the individual and society are more frequent. Conflict is not really the appropriate word, although it well describes many of the interactions between the individual and organized society. Another concept that would have to be employed is discontinuity: the requirement that the individual enter a new situation, learn new things, depart from an accustomed psychological and/or geographical position. The requirement may be perceived as internal or external but in either case the individual frequently (not always) experiences a tension or disjunction implying a temporary or sustained break with the person's accustomed pattern of living. The requirement, be it external or internal, may on the surface appear initially to be, and really be, conflict free. That is to say, it may not be perceived as a requirement at all. For example, if you ask young school children why they go to school, most of them will not say: "I *have* to go to school." "I am *required* to go." Indeed, one of the purposes of socializing young children is to get them to experience going to school as an internal, not an external requirement. It is not

S. B. Sarason, "Individual Psychology: An Obstacle to Comprehending Adulthood," in *Competence and Coping During Adulthood*, ed. L. A. Bond and J. C. Rosen (Hanover, N.H.: University Press of New England, 1980). Copyright 1980 by the Vermont Conference on the Primary Prevention of Psychopathology. Reprinted with permission of University Press of New England.

213

until the middle and high school years that you will find students saying that they are required to go to school. By the time they are adolescents and young adults, most of them know that there are two major types of requirements: the explicit and the implicit, and the implicit has more booby traps. The sense of wariness among young adults that I described in a recent book (Sarason, 1977) is in large measure a reaction to the perception that the abstraction called society would like them to meet a long series of requirements about which they have many doubts. The future may make them feel discontinuous with the present and that may not be desirable. The sense of discontinuity may be in relation to the past or to an imagined future; it may be positively or negatively toned.

Let me use a personal example about a minor discontinuity: me at this conference. George Albee telephones me and invites me to the conference. George cannot require me to attend, but I like and respect George, I have been very impressed with the published proceedings of the previous conferences, and, of course, I am flattered by the invitation. I happen to believe in collegiality and its implication that you have obligations to colleagues to share with them what you think you know, to be disposed to be helpful if they think you can be. The obligations of collegiality involve but go beyond those of courtesy. So, phenomenologically, I had a choice but the fact is that I felt I should want to say yes at the same time I also wanted to say no. I wanted to say no because George was calling me months before the conference and how did I know what life would be like at the end of June, 1978? By age 59 I had learned that making a commitment to the future on the assumption that life is stable, predictable, and controllable is the ultimate in naiveté. For seven years before George called, my wife and I had been taking care of four dying parents. The requirements to do so were both internal and external and, of course, they conflicted with discharging many other types of internal and external requirements. These requirements determined and colored our existence, and, if you like understatements, you can say it was rough. No one likes to feel that planning your life is subject to gross error because you underestimate or ignore possible future requirements and discontinuities to which you will be subject. All of us want to feel that we can control our lives and we invest a lot of energy nurturing the myth of personal freedom, in the process overlooking how in the present we are hemmed in by requirements and, therefore, tending to see the future in similarly unrealistic terms. So, while I was talking to George, I was vaguely aware that if I said yes I would be going against a very strong feeling that I wanted to be free of all requirements, internal or external. "Don't tell me what I can do for you, tell me what you can do for me"—that is one way to describe my view of my world. Two considerations tipped the scales in favor of saying yes. Coming to Burlington would be a break, a way of getting away, however briefly, from an accustomed locale in which I felt bombarded by requirements. Also, my wife might be able to come along and she needed a break no less than I did. It would be a mini-vacation, which can be defined as a sought for, desirable discontinuity. We justify vacations on numerous grounds but surely the need "to get away," "to feel free" from pressures, "to enjoy ourselves" are the most common. When a person says "I want to enjoy myself" that person is saying: "I want only to take myself into account, I want to feel that I am doing something for and only for myself, I do not want to have to take the needs of others into account, I want the experience to be the opposite of what I ordinarily experience." I am no scholar of history but it is my impression that the concept of a vacation as a form of personal indulgence and freedom from a web of requirements is relatively new in human history. The advertisers tell us what we want to hear: our daily lives have a prison-like quality and in order to take it and survive you need to get away from it. There are places you can go to on Eastern's wings of man through United's friendly skies where you can let American do what it does best: take care of every one of *your* needs.

So I go home and tell Esther about lovely Burlington when June is busting out all over. She tells me what I already knew: she has clinical responsibilities until the very end of June and it may not be possible for her to go. My response is that she should stop being so damned conscientious and start giving priorities to her needs, the kind of response that brings smiles to the faces of travel agents and advertisers. It's a short conversation because June is months away and we do not have to make decisions now. Then in February I find myself in the hospital for emergency surgery. That was not a sought for discontinuity! But it was like a lot of other undesirable discontinuities in that it reminded me that I am not the captain of my fate and the master of my soul except within narrower limits than I like to think. However, there was one unintended consequence of the hospitalization and convalescence: nobody required anything of me and everybody was marvelously indulgent of all my presumed needs. Then May rolls around on its way to June. How about it, Esther, are you going to go? I shall not bore you with the protracted negotiations between the two of us. I wish only to state the obvious: each was putting requirements on the other in the course of which each of our views about a desirable discontinuity inevitably changed. Esther and I approach going on any trip in very different ways so that what initially appears will be a conflict free experience always contains elements of conflict. We adjust to each other as much because we feel we have to as because we want to. Neither of us is a free agent. In the meantime I am writing a paper for the conference, furious that I said yes, doubtful that I had anything interesting to say, and feeling quite unfree. Why do I conspire with my world to feel closed in?

If you are a psychologically minded person—and who is not in this age of psychology—my personal account has raised questions in your mind about me as a person. What makes him tick? Why the seemingly dysphoric overtones to what he has recounted? What is his wife like? Why is he so interested in requirements? Are his advancing years getting the better of him? Does he look back with regrets at what he did and did not do? Is he in therapy or should he go into therapy? I can assure you that my purpose in telling you what I did was far more modest and simple than these complicated questions would suggest. My purpose was to suggest that at different times over the course of our lives we are confronted with requirements and discontinuities many of which are predictable but for most of which we are unprepared. And by unprepared I mean that we simply do not think about them, or if we do think about them it is with a large dose of wish fulfillment, or that it is inevitable that the actual experience of these requirements and discontinuities will be different in very important ways from what we imagined. Let me be concrete by telling you some of our interview findings with college seniors making a career choice, with first and fourth year medical students, first and third year law students, and with professionals of varying ages over the life span (Sarason, 1977). In our interview we had a question for those seniors who were going into medicine, law, or some graduate school program, and they represented a clear majority of the seniors. The question was: "Have you ever considered a career in business, finance, or industry?" Their answer was universally an emphatic no and they gave three reasons: you would be a small cog in a big wheel, it takes a long time to get to the top, and the chances are good that you will become morally corrupt in the process. In other words, if you go into medicine and law, you can retain and even develop your individuality and stay true to your idealism. Put in another way, business, finance, and industry are organized on a scale and in ways that require a person to give up something in himself, to accommodate to external requirements, to become unfree. Is it not astounding that these college seniors have divided the world into two parts: one good, and the other evil? How come they know so little about the part of the world they plan to enter: its increasing scale, its structure and organization, its culture, its requirements, its similarities to the "evil" half of the world? How will they experience the discontinuities they seek? When we interviewed medical, law, and graduate students, the picture, of course, changed. Without exception they knew that they were going to be in or around large, bureaucratically organized institutions, small cogs in big wheels, scrambling competitively to get a place in the sun, and quite sensitive to the obstacles to remaining true to their ideals. With some exceptions they look back nostalgically to their good old days and look forward with wariness to the future. Some say explicitly they are disillusioned, others say they are now more "realistic" about the world they are in and will be, no one is unscathed. I do not want to convey the impression that they have become depressives shorn of hope and ambition and dripping with cynicism. What I do wish to convey is that they have been through a series of discontinuous experiences that have left them with a sense of incompleteness and frustration, and with the knowledge that their lives in large measure are and will be determined by forces beyond their control. Most of them by conventional standards have coped well and are competent. By their internal, private standards they have eaten the fruits of worldly knowledge and they are uncertain about how to judge the tastes. Turow's (1977) description of life as a first-year law student at Harvard confirms and deepens the thrust of the conclusions we came to from our interviews, i.e., medical, law, and graduate students would not justify avoiding a career in business, finance, and industry the way they did as seniors.

Now let me tell you about two other groups we have interviewed but have not written up. One is a handful of seniors headed for a career in the arts or the theatre. What is remarkable about them is how crystal clear they are about the obstacles they will confront, and their small chance for success. They are no less idealistic than others, they are no less hopeful that Lady Luck has a special place in her heart for them, but they also know how the "industry" they seek to enter is organized, the disappointments they must be prepared to expect, and how their capacity for self-denial will be tested. They want to be successful but they know they may not be, and they will go on from there. We have not interviewed people like them at different stages of their careers and so we cannot say how they tend to react to obstacles and externally imposed requirements. We can assume that by conventional standards a fair number of people who go into these fields will be "failures" or marginally successful—they did not "make it" and all that implies—but, again, by internal standards the conventional criteria for judging coping and competence may be misleading.

The second group we interviewed consisted of 25 seniors who had majored in the administrative sciences. They were headed for careers in business, finance, and industry. Like the small group of arts and theatre majors, and unlike the premed, prelaw, and pregraduate school seniors, they seemed to have an appreciation of the characteristics of the organizations in which they planned to work. Here again these students had their ambitions and ideals and knew that their working days would not be without their conflicts, frustrations, and moral-testing experiences. But, they felt, there would be challenges and opportunities for creativity. They too were wary but they felt they knew what they were getting in to.

There were two other groups I have known well over the years: teachers in training, and experienced teachers seeking credentials to become administrators. I have discussed the training and education of these groups in detail elsewhere (Sarason, 1971) and so let it suffice for my present purposes to say that when they begin their careers, they are remarkably unknowledgeable about the culture, organization, and traditions of a school and a school system. Years ago some colleagues and I (Sarason, Davidson, and Blatt, 1962) wrote a book titled *The Preparation of Teachers. An Unstudied Problem in Education.* The theme of the book was that the preparation of teachers ill prepared them to understand a classroom, let along the cultural-structural dynamics of a school and school system. The book went into oblivion rather quickly and our only solace is that what later happened in the sixties confirmed in spades what we had said. That practically nobody (really nobody) took us seriously should not have surprised us. After all, we were suggesting that the conventional criteria by which coping and competence were being judged were inadequate and no one knew this better than teachers and school administrators who, of course, were not about to make the truth public.

Now let me state some similarities between what I have described about these groups (with the exception of the administrative science and theatre majors) and what I said about me and the conference.

I was not well prepared for the discontinuities I experienced in connection with taking care of old parents. My world was structured around family and work and that structure had a future thrust to it and a content to which I looked forward. I was, of course, aware that our parents lived elsewhere, they were obviously aging, and that we would have to be prepared for their increasing dependence on us. But that knowledge was of a hazy sort containing a large dose of wish fulfillment. We would handle matters as they came up. What we did not know, but could have known, was that when old people become sick and dependent, they and you have to deal with a part of our society that has structure and traditions which, if you do not understand and know how to cope with, can make life difficult indeed. No less significant is the effect of coping (with doctors, hospitals, nursing homes, home care aides, medicare, social service agencies) on the structure and functioning of your family and work worlds. It is not that you become aware of how these worlds have become interrelated but rather that you are no longer as free as you were and the future is now suffused with oppressiveness and anxiety. Planning a future becomes a kind of luxury as you find yourself caught in a web of requirements, wondering how long you can or should take it, torn between feelings of anger and compassion, hardly able to control rage against "them": against everybody who expects you to conform to their needs and rules. What I have just related about myself I have gotten from several medical, law, and graduate students. These were extreme cases but I can assure you that a lot of interviewees reported the feeling of being unprepared, of having had their eyes opened to the culture and structure of the setting they were in. Here again I must caution you not to conclude that these students were in a state of shock, unable to cope and to be competent. All that I am saying is that they have varying degrees of disillusionment and disappointment about how their working world is structured so that they are less certain than before that they are in control of their lives. And they perceive a sharp break between their past and present lives. For the bulk of them there is a poignant moral dilemma. How can they survive in the structures they are embedded in and not "sell out"? How will they know when they are being brainwashed? Will they ever really be free to go their own way?

Another story. A Yale student, headed for graduate school in psychology, worked with me for a year and when we parted for the summer we agreed to meet in the fall about what schools he should consider. When we met in the fall, he told me his plans had changed and he wanted to go to medical school. He had gotten a job that summer in a large general hospital and he was aghast at the impersonal treatment patients received, the small amount of time physicians gave to patients, the view of patients as objects rather than people, and the psychological insensitivity of medical personnel. Larry wanted to become a general practitioner who would really treat his patients the way they deserved and needed to be treated. He was a bright, creative, hard-working young man prepared to devote his life to others. I listened, my heart sank, and I did something I never did before. I tried to dissuade him. I described in detail what medical school was like, its structure, the formal and informal hierarchy of values by which students are judged, the financial indebtedness he would incur (he was not a rich boy) over a seven-year period of training, what this would mean for his love life (he had a girl friend), the costs of set-

220 SEYMOUR B. SARASON

ting up and sustaining a practice, and how time will become money and what that means for how much time you can give a patient. I concluded by saying: "to be with patients the way you want, to charge them fees they can afford, to treat them not according to the clock or the number of patients in the waiting room means that you will have to be satisfied to live on $30,000 or $40,000 a year. That sounds like a lot to you now but after years of training and indebtedness, and hopefully after marriage and children, is that income likely to be satisfactory?" Larry was not disposed to listen. He applied to medical school, got in, but I have never heard from him. I hope I was wrong in my forecast. Our interviews suggest that I stand a chance of having been correct. Incidentally, lest you think that I am picking on physicians, or medical schools, or the culture and structure of American medicine, I should tell you that I was prepared to discuss with Larry what graduate school in psychology would be like and my speech would in principle have been similar to the one I gave to him.

All that I have so far said leads to a conclusion crucial to how one thinks about coping and competence in adulthood. But before stating that conclusion, and as a way of helping you grasp its significances, I will describe to you what I now do in my seminars all of which have to do with structural-cultural features of our society. I present them in the very first meeting with the following task:

There are two kinds of people here: Yale seniors and graduate students from different departments. You have all experienced several years of living in a university. Now this seminar is not about universities but about other kinds of institutions: public schools, mental hospitals, correctional facilities, institutions for the retarded, human services agencies and the like. Our focus will be on how these institutions have changed over time and how we think they ought to change in the future. But if you want to change these institutions, you have to try to understand them. I can safely assume that you have little or no knowledge of or experience with these institutions. I can also assume that you feel that you are ignorant with respect to them, that there is nothing in your experience which would permit you to say that even though you may never have set foot in them, you know something about them. I suggest that you do know, or could relatively quickly know, some important things about these institutions based on your past experience with the university. To prove this to you I want you to take the next half hour and answer these questions:

1. How many schools does Yale (or any other university) consist of? What are the administrative relationships among these schools?
2. Describe the procedures by which a university grants tenure to a faculty member. When does the procedure begin, who participates

when, what information is sought, when, and from whom, when is the decision final, and why are some people granted tenure and others are not?

3. How are departmental chairmen chosen, what are their responsibilities and formal powers, and how do they relate to higher levels of administration?

4. You have had many dealings with individual faculty members, deans, and other staff. How would you characterize these dealings? Were they helpful, instructive? If not, how do you explain it? Do you feel the university exists for you, the alumni, the faculty?

The exercise serves two major purposes. First, it impresses on the students the fact, surprising to them, that although they have been living in the university for several years, they are amazingly ignorant of its structure, functions, and practices. In their interactions with different people and parts of the university they form impressions and opinions about the university but they are unable to place those interactions other than in an individual framework. Their explanations of how they have been influenced by their university experiences are psychological in nature, and they are almost wholly unable to take distance from themselves and to try to see the hows and whys of organizational structure, dynamics, and functions. And when I say "wholly unable" I mean that in the normal course of living they feel no particular need to describe and understand the characteristics of the large organizational picture in which they are embedded. They are, for example, interested in how Yale selects students and the consequences of that selection process for their lives at Yale. But they are far less interested in how faculty are selected, even though they know how they are being affected by the faculty whom they see as bewilderingly varied.

The second purpose of the exercise is for me to help them understand better the university's organizational character which impacts their lives in countless important ways even though they are ordinarily unaware of it. Just as the architecture of a house or building has psychological consequences for its inhabitants, so do the organizational traditions and structure of the the university affect the lives of all of its inhabitants. The point I try to impress on the students is that you can *see* people, *you cannot see an organization and its structure.* If you want to understand a setting, you cannot restrict yourself literally to seeing it. You must have a set of concepts that allow you to go beyond the concrete, the palpable, the percept. So, I ask them, how many of you see the faculty as consisting of individuals each of whom seems to be absorbed in what he or she considers important? How many of you have noticed how rare it is for faculty members to work with each other? The answer to the first question is an emphatic yes; to the second question the answer is that it is rare. How should we go about trying to understand what we see? We discuss many things among which is a factor I stumbled on one day after 25 years at Yale. That I stumbled on it then is important because it came at a time 10 years ago when I was trying to understand why I experienced my adulthood in the ways I did. My explanations had been primarily, but not exclusively, psychological: I was a certain kind of person, and "they" were different kinds of people; I had certain needs, assets, and vulnerabilities that tended to clash with those of "them." Needless to say, I was responding to them and me as individuals, and whatever clashes had occurred, to put it neutrally, were due to individual differences. Then the clouds parted and some light came through in the form of two questions: Who tries to make it in the university? Whom does the university select? The answer to both questions is rugged individualism. So you have a selection process that gives you assertive, ambitious, prima donna types and then you wonder why they go their own way and frequently clash. You need more than psychology to understand faculty behavior.

I am of the opinion that adulthood cannot be productively understood in terms of psychology, at least the psychologies that are currently dominant. Paradoxically, they suffer from the defect of their virtue: the attempt to rivet on the development of internal structure and organization. Freud, Paiget, the Gestaltists, and their descendants, focussed on the individual psyche, what Murray Levine calls the emphasis on "intrapsychic supremacy." In no way do I wish to derogate their contributions and influences. But it needs to be recognized that their pioneering efforts to conceptualize internal content, structure, and organization were at the expense of doing justice to the fact that we are born into and live out our lives in a variety of contexts possessing structure and organization no less fateful than those of our psyches. (Freud understood this in small measure in terms of family structure and organization.)

When I try to make sense of my adult years, and when I reflect on the many interviews we conducted with people at different points in adulthood, I come to the conclusion that adulthood is that long period of our lives in which we learn that every part of our individual worlds, every experience, reflects two kinds of impact: our impact on an existing external structure and organization, and the impact of that external structure and organization on us. I deliberately do not use the term environment because it is too global and too easily distracts us from the crucial characteristics of structure and organization.

Whether we are in an aeroplane, a classroom, a faculty meeting, at the dinner table, at a conference, or in a new work setting, our experience is not understandable without seeing it in relation to the structure, organization, and traditions of the setting. That may seem obvious to you but my experience and research suggests that we have an amazing capacity to ignore the obvious. We are psychologically minded not structure-organizationally minded.

Adulthood has become increasingly problematic for many people as they find that in all spheres of living they are part of organized, complex structures they neither understand nor can change. It would be more correct to say that their understanding is so personal, so psychological, that they are cut off from ways of thinking and acting that might be more effective. No less important, they cannot entertain the possibility that what they have experienced is generalizable to many other structured settings. So, the students in my seminars have difficulty with the idea that if they understood the structure and organization of Yale, and how it has directly and indirectly shaped their lives, they would know a lot about life in seemingly very different settings. This is not to say, of course, that Yale is the same as these other institutions but rather that all of them—by virtue of being complex, structured, hierarchically organized, historical settings in a society like ours—will present similar problems to those who live in these settings. The similarities have little or nothing to do with personalities but far more with the history and traditions of the society in which these settings evolved.

When I compare college freshmen with college seniors; college seniors with first-year law, medical and graduate students; these first-year students with those finishing professional and graduate schools; and all of these groups with people who have been full fledged professionals for varying periods of time, I am forced to the conclusion that adulthood is a continuous process during which blinders become removed from the eyes of individuals as they are forced to recognize that far from being free individuals they are always part of and restricted by a social matrix. They do become more structure-organizationally minded but, more often than not, it is with reluctance or bitterness or resignation. Some of them reach the understanding that what they have learned about how our society is structured and organized was new to them but that it has been true of our society for a long time. Many people take it far more personally, as if it was all arranged to defeat them.

Prior to World War II our country was self-consciously and deliberately isolationist. We wanted to involve ourselves as little as possible in the intanglements overseas. We viewed ourselves as self-sufficient as a country could be: protected by two oceans and possessed of boundless resources. We recognized that there were other societies but their problems were their problems and we should not allow ourselves to be affected by what they did. Now we know how shortsighted, self-defeating, and ignorant we were of the forces that had been let loose on this earth. We had to be hit over the head to force us to recognize that we were part of this world, like it or not. For the most part we have not liked it because we are so new at understanding and dealing with how this world is organized, puzzled by our increasing dependence on others, angry at finding ourselves in a web we did not weave, regretful that we were not better prepared for our adulthood as a nation. Analogously, that is the way many people today look on their individual adulthoods. And that is why so many of them seek new life styles or new places in an attempt to escape from their social web. Some of them fail because they still need to believe that they can be independent of social webs, i.e., that one can weave one's own web independent of the webs of all other people. Some succeed in the sense that they do not deny the facts of social living in our society but use their new understanding to strike a better compromise between internal needs and external structures. This new understanding, I have to emphasize, is only in part psychological in the narrow sense. This new understanding is in large part based on new knowledge about external structures.

World War II ushered in the Age of Psychology, some would say the Age of Mental Health. As individuals we were interested in ourselves, and so were myriad professionals eager to tell us how to understand ourselves. I should not use the past tense because this new age is still with us, flourishing and spawning a thriving industry. It is an industry that is providing people with what they feel they need. But it is also an industry that unwittingly colludes with its consumers in believing that the locus of trouble in people is within them. There is, of course, passing recognition that the troubles are somehow related to our social context that confine and frustrate us and seem to become interrelated over time. The problem, as someone once put it, is: how do you stay sane in an insane world? The question implies that there is little point in trying to understand the world and if you make the effort, you will end up more convinced than ever that the less you have to do with the world the better. But the world is not insane, and we must be careful to avoid the error of using a psychology of the individual to understand how and why our worlds are structured as they are. Society is not a random collection of entities and forces. It did not take the shape it did for the hell of it. We may not like that shape but surely we cannot be content only with aesthetic judgment because, if we are, we can never glimpse how and why that shape evolved and is still evolving.

Permit me to make one more effort to illustrate the unfortunate consequences of looking at persons, any person, from our customary focus on individuals. As you will see, these consequences are no less unfortunate when we look at *an* organization or setting as we do individuals. Take the film *One Flew Over the Cuckoo's Nest,* whose locale is a mental hospital. We are not concerned here with the artistic quality of the film, but rather with the major themes it conveys. The first is that there is an *interpersonal* struggle between two very dominant and assertive people. A second theme is that the struggle is not only between two people of unequal status and power but that the *personality* of each is lethal to the other. A third theme is that the patient-hero is fated to lose in his battle against *officialdom of the hospital.* There are other more muted or less articulated themes (e.g., the ward patients are "sick" people who need and even want hospitalization; doubt is raised about the therapeutic value of the hospital but if these patients were to leave, as they do *en masse* at one point, they would prove they were indeed sick people from whom the community needed protection as the patients need protection against themselves). It is hard to avoid coming away from the film without feeling that if either of the two protagonists had been different, tragedy would have been avoided. In short, it is a drama of individuals.

We did an informal study. Whenever we met social scientists, we asked them how they reacted to the film. Almost without exception they said they liked the picture, i.e., it was a moving and involving, although upsetting, experience. Why was it upsetting? By far the most frequent answer was in terms of people's inhumanity to other people, witting or unwitting. As one put it: "If that nurse had not been stupid, insensitive, and rigid, there would be no point to the film." Or as another said: "It is frightening to see how power can be abused." The next most frequent answer was the expressions of puzzlement: granted that the nurse was a hateful creature, how do you deal with such an assortment of crazy people? One person said: "I suppose a hospital like that brings out the worst in everybody." Not one of these social scientists showed the slightest recognition that this mental hospital was part of a state system of mental health services having a central office staffed with professionals who have policy making and policy implementing functions, the scope of which is in part a reflection of policies and arrangements arrived at through the political process involving the executive and legislative branches of government; and that all of the foregoing is tied in with and affected by federal policies and grant support, and in the formation of these federal policies mental health professionals play an important but not an exclusive role. But what is the relevance of this to their reactions to the film? There are two ways of answering—one general and one specific. The general answer is that the study of public policy rests on, among other things, the assumption that any particualr policy (e.g., energy) will have consequences for more than one system or sector in society (e.g., public utilities, automobiles), and that the policy always reflects political and economic factors. Put in another way: when an energy policy (federal and state) was developed, it altered the thinking and planning of countless individual agencies and organizations. Or, when the federal or state governments change their welfare policy, there are consequences not only for the welfare "system" but for many other systems as well. Indeed, perhaps the most troublesome task in policy reconstruction, analysis, and formulation is in understanding effects on interacting systems. But for our purposes one can disregard the fact of interacting systems and still make the important, if obvious, point that a public policy in regard to one system affects all parts of that system, and no one part can be understood in terms only of itself. The mental hospital in the film was part of a system and one cannot understand that hospital unless one sees it in terms of its embeddedness in that system. The specific part of the answer concerns the last part of the film when we see McMurphy, the patient-hero, electroshocked into submission and senselessness. All to whom we spoke found themselves shuddering at these scenes. Some thought it brutal, period. Some thought it brutal but were bothered by the question: What do you do with a McMurphy? Some people equated the brutality with conscious sadism, but most people viewed it more as institutionalized stupidity and insensitivity in the service of institutional law and order. *However, if the general answer above has validity, then this part of the film cannot be understood only in terms of that hospital and its personnel.* For example, most of the film takes place in a ward, but for all practical purposes a psychiatrist is never there. This, of course, is not happenstance. That is the case in almost every mental hospital. It is beyond the scope of this paper to pursue this matter except to say that it cannot be understood apart from the resources available to the state and federal hospital system and the consequences for hospital organization and functioning, e.g., what kinds of people will be hired, to whom responsibility will be given, the kinds of treatment to be employed, the development and maintenance of community placements, criteria for admission and discharge. The state hospital, far from being autonomous, must function in conformity with a system. No one know this better than hospital employees, professional or otherwise. Just like urban teachers see their problems in large part in terms of "downtown," hospital staff similarly look to "the central office" in the capitol, who in turn look to the state executive and legislative branches, who in turn look to "Washington" as insensitive, penurious, and capricious. If you think of the hospital as a person, you can say that just as in the film McMurphy was electroshocked into conformity, the hospital feels that in countless ways it is forced to conform to "the system." To try to understand what a mental hospital is by studying *it* is conceptually nonsensical; it is the kind of nonsense that has the unintended effect of making sure that immorality will flourish.

To comprehend adulthood in our times and in the foreseeable future we have to look at two factors. The first is that we have become a psychologically minded society. Self actualization, self realization, human potential, and self expression have become household phrases. The psychotherapies in their myriad forms are available to almost everyone. Know thyself has, twenty-five hundred years after Socrates, been incorporated in public policy and insurance policies. And in the controversies that have swirled around the field of public education, the only point of agreement is that each child should realize his full potential, i.e., to make him aware of and to help him develop his capacities. All of this has become so familiar, so much a part of our way of thinking, that to question any of it on any basis is to run the risk of being considered stupid, obtuse, and obviously in need of deeper self-knowledge. From a theoretical and technical standpoint, the major questions have become: how can we help everyone get to know themselves better? What is the best and quickest way to do that: by therapies that deal with one's past or by those that focus on the here and now? And which of several scores of professions should be empowered to help or teach us to know ourselves better? But although each of these therapies deal with individuals who have problems, each of them is based on an implicit or explicit conception of how you can prevent problems, and, very briefly but not surprising, that conception centers around individual characteristics and patterns of abilities.

This emphasis on a psychology of the individual, long a characteristic of American psychology but never so clear as in the post World War II period, is matched in its pervasiveness by a feature of western society that for all practical purposes this individual psychology has ignored. I refer to the fact that the organizations in which we live our lives are bigger, more bureaucratic, more interconnected among themselves, less autonomous, more subject to centralized government control, and more vulnerable to international economic dynamics than ever before. I am not making or implying a political judgment. I am saying something all of you sense: when you turn your attention away from yourself and have to look at and deal with the structure of and interconnections among organizations, it is as if you are dealing with wheels within wheels, i.e., everything seems to have become related to everything else. When I say related, I do not mean that the relationships are understandable in terms of cause and effect or that their functional relationships are the result of rational planning. On the contrary, the reverse is true. All that we feel secure about is that at the same time that we seem to feel everything is related to everything else, we also feel that disorganization is increasing. At the same time that we say that individuals suffer from loneliness, anomie, isolation, and unconnectedness, the external world—the world of societal organizations and structures—is on the road to greater connectedness and interpenetration.

It is beyond the scope of this paper to attempt to explain these two factors that are so characteristic of our times. It is, however, central to my purpose to emphasize that adulthood has become psychologically problematic, in large measure because so many people come to and live through adulthood without ways for understanding the nature and thrust of the world of social organization. The two factors have been on a collision course. When young adults go out into the real world, they are not aware they have been living in the real world. From the time they enter school as young children to the time they leave college or postgraduate schools as adults, they have been living in complex organizations, but they learn little or nothing about these organizations *qua* organizations. They are taught a lot of things, but not about how their parochial context of learning bears the stamp of larger, interconnected organizational structures. So, when they finish schooling and are catapulted into the larger society, many of them are jolted by the experience because they simply do not have schemas by which to accomodate to and assimilate what they are experiencing. Of course they accomodate and assimilate but if you are partisan to a Piagetian way of viewing things, you would never conclude that they understand the structure of the social world. The reverence for Piaget is explainable on three grounds. First, he brilliantly clarified the development of logical thinking in relation to the perceptible world. Second, his contributions fitted smoothly into an individual psychology. And third, they were, so to speak, tailor-made for an age that believed in science as the means by which all major societal problems would ultimately be solved. As Piaget's star was reaching its zenith, hundreds of people began to explore how his findings and ideas could be incorporated into education with the goal, of course, of better preparing people for adulthood, i.e., if you want to prepare more competent people for adulthood, then Piaget had given us a good part of the answer. Not that the aim was to prepare everyone to become logicians or scientists, but rather to insure that they would end up with the schemas by which they would be able more effectively to comprehend and cope with their world. Unfortunately, none of these people was asking what that world was. What aspect of the world were they talking about? The world as anthropologists may see it? As political scientists may see it? As sociologists may see it? And the head of a task force on governmental reorganization may see it?

Our knowledge of the atom would not have gone much beyond that of the Greeks if along the way people had not begun to make the assumption that the atom had structure. What was that structure and how can we get to know it, was what people began to ask. And how is that structure related to or manifested in other types of structures in the imperceptible world? Could we control, manipulate, exploit these structures? Analogous questions are asked by people throughout their adulthood about their social world. But unlike the atomic scientist, adults ask questions about their social world less out of curiosity and more because they feel forced to for the purposes of sanity and survival. Some stop asking questions, however early they may have reached the highest levels of logical thinking. Some, and again, independent of their level of logical or scientific thinking, accommodate to perplexities about their social world by assimilating, child-like, theories that explain everything. Most people, I would guess, and especially because what they know about the larger society comes from television and movies, change their explanations in fad-like fashion. Elsewhere (1978) I have discussed the interesting case of the atomic scientists who, at the very moment they were at the apogee of public respect and acclaim because they had learned to control nuclear processes and successfully explode a bomb, experienced a massive disillusionment when their efforts to influence public policy in certain ways were rebuffed. Like so many young adults, these sophisticated scientists were babes in the woods of societal structures, institutions, and traditions. They were eating some new species of the fruits of knowledge and the taste was not to their liking.

I trust that no one here believes that you can or should try to make the experience of adulthood as unproblematic as possible. Such a goal would reflect the most profound ignorance of what societies have been, are, and will be. It is a goal no less illusory than the belief that the phenomenology of living can be uninformed by the knowledge of our mortality. To the extent that we view and study adulthood in terms of our current psychologies that are so riveted on the individual we will be wasting time and, perhaps, causing more harm than good because we will be reinforcing the mistaken belief that you can know yourself without knowing your society, that you can know your changing self without knowing your changing society.

Just as parents' relationships to a child begin before the child is born, an adult's conception of his adulthood begins long before he has met society's definition of adulthood. And in those early preschool years those messages children receive, we adults know, contain a lot of myth. (Yes, Virginia, there is a Santa Claus.) I have no strong objections to these myths and I have no desire to make young children worldly philosophers. But I do object to the belief that as children acquire a formal and informal education, they will have gotten an understanding of the "real world" that will permit them in adulthood to be competent in that world. From my standpoint, competence is more than successfully competing, or utilizing one's capacities effectively, or being able to change adaptively to new circumstances, or deepening one's knowledge of self. The missing ingredient is how well we persist with the effort to deepen our understanding of the fact that we are embedded in and expressions of a near and distant social world. Without that missing ingredient we are perilously close to defining human and subhuman competence by the same criteria, with the exception, of course, of deepening one's knowledge of self. But that is my point: as soon as you include deepening one's knowledge of one's self you imply that the validity of such knowledge can be determined independent of one's understanding of how what one does, think, and concludes always reflects embeddedness in a near and distant social world. If my personal life is any guide, and my work with people at different points in adulthood encourages me that I am not very atypical, the missing ingredient forces itself into our thinking as we learn how naive we were about the structure, forces, and underpinnings of our near and distant social worlds. Why was that ingredient missing earlier in our lives? Or, if it was not missing, why was our understanding so wrong?

If we are different from subhumans it is in our potential to comprehend ourselves in relation to the natural world and the social world We have done well with respect to the natural world although it could be argued that our ignorance about the social world permitted the advances of science to transform the social world in ways inimical to human existence or, at the very least, to make comprehending the social world extraordinarily difficult because it has made the interconnectedness of the social world so difficult to experience and comprehend. In any event, the social world will become more interconnected and complex, we will increasingly be affected by it, and, it may be, we will continue to conceptualize and deal with it in narrow psychological terms. If we continue in our enamorment with the psychology of the individual, it will be a monument to trivialization. And if when we talk about prevention of the disabilities that can occur in adulthood, we restrict ourselves to their prevention in individuals, our efforts are doomed. I am not a Marxist, although I was when I entered adulthood because I thought it explained to me how society was organized, where it was going, and a good deal about myself. Marx, and especially the Marxists that came after him, were, at best, incomplete, wrong, and misguided in their thinking, and, at worst, witting and unwitting perpetrators of social catastrophes. But, I must emphasize, Marx was dealing with the most important problem: the relationship between how people think and the structure and dynamics of the social world. And he was right when he said that the task is not only to understand this relationship but to change it. I am not making a political statement or calling for political action. At this point I would appreciate a little more understanding and less misplaced emphasis.

REFERENCES

Sarason, Seymour B. *The Culture of the School and the Problem of Change.* Boston: Allyn & Bacon, 1971.

Sarason, Seymour B. *Work, Aging, and Social Change. Professionals and the One Life-One Career Imperative.* New York: Free Press, 1977.

Sarason, Seymour B. "The Nature of Problem Solving in Social Action." *American Psychologist*, April 1978, Vol. 33, No. 4, pp. 370–380.

Sarason, Seymour B., Kenneth S. Davidson, and Burton Blatt. *The Preparation of Teachers. An Unstudied Problem in Education.* New York: John Wiley, 1962.

Turow, Scott. *One L.* New York: Putnam, 1977.

Commentary to
Chapter 15

*This paper was my presidential address in 1980 to the Division of
Clinical Psychology of the American Psychological Association. In it
I explain why I believe that the tie forged between clinical psychology
and medical-psychiatric settings was a major mistake for psychology
generally and clinical psychology in particular. How and why did
these ties get forged shortly after World War II? What other alternatives could or did psychology consider in its desire to deal with pres-
sing social problems that affect individual lives? Why had clinical
psychology become no less exclusive and professionally precious
than psychiatry? I was aware that people coming into clinical psychology are abysmally ignorant of the origins of modern clinical
psychology. They are unaware that what they think about as clinicians, where they think about it, and the interprofessional conflicts
they experience stem directly from a series of actions during and
immediately after World War II. I did not write this address, however,
only to give glimpses of how the past is in the present and again to criticize psychology's ahistorical stance. What I wanted to demonstrate,
more concretely than I had done in any previous paper, is how psychology's dependence on an individual psychology provides a misleading foundation for thinking about psychology's relation to
society, government, and the medical setting.*

*It is obvious from my previous papers that I believed that psy-
chology was (and continues to be) ill prepared to deal with policies
and issues directly reflecting the nature of our society. First, psychology, and therefore psychological theory, was never self-conscious
about how it reflected the society. In addition, psychological theory
and research, whatever their virtues, never directed themselves to
how the society was ordered; the social-historical matrix from which
that social order emerged; the political, legislative, and judicial institutions that bulwarked the social order—how it came about that an
enormous change had taken place in the strength and scope of the
federal government; and, fatefully, the pluses and minuses that this
change brought in its wake. It might be argued that I am criticizing
psychology for not studying everything and not knowing everything. That would be a cogent response if psychology had remained,
as it was in the pre–World War II period, a minuscule, laboratory-*

oriented field housed in the university. The fact is that, after the war, psychology sought to play a significant role in relation to society's problems. Psychology did not come kicking and screaming into the arena of governmental policy, nor did it have reservations about why it was sought out to be an object as well as an instrumentality of public policy. Nothing illustrates the limitations of American psychology as clearly as the story of how modern clinical psychology took on the features it did. With the best of intentions, and with an amazingly naive understanding of American society in general and the culture of American medicine, psychology exposed its ignorance of the society of which it was a part.

Almost everything I say in this paper I said thirty years ago, with no less conviction, although I now understand what happened in a more conceptual and less personal way. I take no satisfaction in having been right, because, as the years went by, my disenchantment with what was happening to clinical psychology strained relationships with people I liked and led to frequent feelings of marginality and isolation, which I would have preferred not to have experienced. What does give me satisfaction is the substance of the most frequent response to the address: "I am glad you said out loud what I and others think." If anybody ever asked me wherein my thinking has any distinctiveness, I would say that it was in taking the obvious seriously. American psychology has had trouble recognizing the obvious, perhaps because so much attention has been given to the distractions of theory.

15

An Asocial Psychology and a Misdirected Clinical Psychology

In what social-historical context did the major features of modern clinical psychology initially gain expression? How did this context affect the universe of policy alternatives modern clinical psychology could have considered in its early phase? Why did clinical psychology so readily accommodate to a public policy that not only defined what the "mental health problem" was in our society but also outlined how that problem was to be approached? And why did the basis of that approach in an individual psychology go unexamined? It is the last question that interests me the most because I have come to believe that from its inception a hundred years ago, American psychology has been quintessentially a psychology of the individual organism, a characteristic that however it may have been and is productive has severely and adversely affected psychology's contribution to human welfare. I elaborate later on this point, but those who may want to delve more deeply into this question I urge to read the APA publication edited by Hilgard (1978), which contains addresses of presidents of the association, beginning with William James. With one notable exception one would hardly know that psychology existed in a particular society having a distinctive social order deriving from a very distinctive past, that psychologists did not (and do not) represent a random assortment of people, and that by virtue of their socialization into their society, and their social-

S. B. Sarason, "An Asocial Psychology and a Misdirected Clinical Psychology," *American Psychologist* 36 (8): 827–836. Copyright 1981 by the American Psychological Association. Reprinted by permission. This article was originally the presidential address to Division 12 (Clinical Psychology), presented at the meeting of the American Psychological Association, Montrial, September 1980. The author gratefully acknowledges the help provided by Michael Klaber during the writing of this article.

professional niche in it, the *substance* of their theories had to reflect these factors. Instead, one finds a riveting on the individual organism. The one notable exception, and it is a dramatically instructive exception, is a presidential address given in 1899 in New Haven with the title "Psychology and Social Practice." If psychology (then and now) had been able to understand this address, which was quite critical of the directions psychology was taking, American psychology would not now be suffering the malaise it is.

I have recently completed a book, *Psychology Misdirected* (Sarason, 1981), that is dedicated to the APA president who gave that address: John Dewey. Psychologists think of John Dewey, when they think of him at all, as an educator and philosopher who *once* was a psychologist. But Dewey saw clearly what psychology still is blind to: The substance of psychology cannot be independent of the social order. It is not that it *should not* be independent but that it *cannot* be. But American psychology has never felt comfortable pursuing the nature and consequences of the social order. Let the other social sciences wrestle with such matters! Besides, a true understanding of the social order, as well as efforts to change and improve it, could only come after psychology illuminated human nature, individual human nature. Psychology had it backwards, a fact to which it cannot be sensitive as long as theories are about individuals—as single individuals, as individuals in a dyad or small group, or as individuals in a family. For all practical purposes, social history and the social order were ignored. And this explains why when psychology really entered the "real world" and the arena of public policy in the post-World War II period, it was, from my standpoint, the beginning of a disaster. I must now turn to elaborating on these points by reflecting on the history of modern clinical psychology. This introduction has been necessary if only to underline the point that the limitations of clinical psychology inhered in American psychology.

CONSEQUENCES OF WORLD WAR II

Modern clinical psychology was a direct outgrowth of World War II. At all levels of federal government during the war, there was recognition that the government would have responsibility for a staggering number of veterans who in one way or another would be physical or mental casualties. That the government "owed" these casualties the best kind of care was clear, and the best kind of care would have to be quite different from that provided veterans in the decades after World War I. To provide this care would require a policy that would facilitate the placement of facilities and services in or near medical centers. That policy was intended to create a partnership between the Veterans Administration (VA) and the medical centers, the bulk of which would be university based. The VA wanted the quality services the medical centers could provide, and the medical centers needed the new facilities for training and research. No one raised the possibility that given the traditions of medical centers, especially their professional preciousness and imperialistic ambience, partnership would, in practice, mean domination by the medical centers. It was a policy that assumed that self-serving professionalism would not be a problem. It was not a policy rooted in the sociology of professions in general and the medical profession in particular. Indeed (as I discuss later in relation to clinical psychology), one of the characteristics of the policymaking process is the absence of sensitivity to social history. But there was an even more fateful, implicit assumption to the policy: Veterans would get "better" in the hospitals and clinics and then return to their homes and communities. That assumption contains a kernel of truth in relation to physical illness, but if I had the time I would have no difficulty demonstrating that from the standpoint of prevention of personal, family, and work problems, this kernel of truth is not all that impressive. In relation to psychological problems there is no kernel of truth. By their very nature these probems are individual–family–work–community related. In fact, as the VA learned in subsequent decades, hospitalization and clinic visits that focused on the intrapsychic dynamics of the individual were frequently counterproductive or simply ineffective.

Another important stimulus to the formulation of a policy for casualties of the war was an economic one, not only in terms of money for facilities and personnel but in terms of payments to veterans depending on their degree of war-incurred handicap. I am not attributing unworthy motivations to the policymakers when I say they were quite concerned that many veterans would seek to obtain payments from the government disproportionate to their handicaps and that some would manufacture symptoms to be eligible for payments. In short, there was the potential for an adversary relationship between the veterans and the professionals in the medical centers who would have to render judgments about degree of disability. This, of course, raised the question, Whom did the professionals represent? The potential for conflicts of interests, as well as for self-serving actions, was obvious on all sides. If what was obvious was not taken seriously, it was in part because everyone assumed that money would not be a problem, that the VA budget would increase to meet needs. So what if some veterans were getting benefits they did not merit? It may be somewhat unfair to say that the policymakers envisioned an endless gravy train. It is not unfair to say that they were naively ahistorical in the extreme in adopting such a stance toward the future. It took less than a decade for the professionals to learn that they were enmeshed in a system which put serious obstacles in the way of their therapeutic efforts and raised ethical–moral questions the professionals did not know how to deal with, except by getting out, which many began to do.

Unless one lived through those early post-World War II days, it is hard to appreciate the role of money as an incentive to medical center departments to enter the partnership. In the case of psychiatry, which up to World War II was not a strong or prestigeful part of medical schools and medical centers, the VA presented a fairyland of delights: new facilities, additional personnel, residencies paid for by the government, consulting fees for faculty, research budgets, and all else that makes for gracious living. There are no grounds for questioning the sincerity of departments of psychiatry insofar as helping veterans was concerned. There are grounds for saying that the VA medical center tie presented psychiatry with the opportunity to become more influential vis-à-vis other specialties. And it is also true that departments of psychiatry did not see this tie as an end in itself but as a means whereby other non-VA activities were made possible. Noblesse oblige characterized psychiatry's stance, which in practice meant, as it does in some legal partnerships, that there was a general partner and a limited partner. Guess who was the limited partner? The economics of the VA medical center tie reinforced the imperialistic traditions of American medicine, resulting in battles among medical departments and in "foreign" wars with "allied" health fields centering around resources, status, and prerogatives.

One could ask me, "Assuming you are even partially correct—about not getting 'better' in a hospital or clinic; about the consequences of personal troubles for family, community, and work; about the self-serving actions that money (a lot of it!) as an incentive played into—why didn't the policymakers know these things? Did they know them but in examining alternative policies find none that had fewer pitfalls?" To answer these questions requires that one ask and answer the question, Who were the policymakers? In a formal, flow chart, descriptive sense this is not an easy question to answer but in terms of informal process and power the answer is clear: The "official," legislatively sanctioned policymakers were mightily influenced by representatives of university medical centers who were in high positions in the armed forces during World War II or who were called in as consultants. Their sincerity was as unquestioned as their ability to dispassionately consider alternatives was lacking. On the surface it might seem that their support for a VA–medical center relationship was blatantly self-serving; after all, they were advocating a policy that would pour millions of dollars into their institutions. The self-serving feature was there, but it should not obscure the fact that academic psychiatry saw itself at the threshold of a new era, as leaving behind the aridities, superficialities, and sterile biologisms of prewar psychiatry for a new psychiatry that was "dynamic," "deep," and effective. Psychoanalysis became legitimated by academic psychiatry, which meant that the analytic-training institutes—religious in attitude and ritual, desperate to become a recognized medical specialty, uncomfortable and silent about Freud's position on lay analysis, and disdainful of those who did not accept Freud's truths as interpreted by institute-anointed ayatollahs—added an ingredient quite compatible with the medical profession's attitudes of preciousness, exclusiveness, special social status, and tradition-conferred leadership role.

All that I have said so far can be summarized as follows: Health policy for veterans, formulated in terms of medical concepts, practices, and traditions, sought to interrelate two organizational cultures—the university medical center and a large, complex federal bureau. Neither of the organizations had experience with such a formal interrelationship, and neither attempted to understand the other's culture and what that presaged for their future relationships. It was a policy that stemmed from a process amazingly devoid of serious consideration of alternative approaches; it was a medical policy in terms of who would be responsible for implementation and what the nature (and language) and where the site of diagnosis and treatment would be.

Concern and responsibility for veterans was only one of the ingredients that helped usher in the new Age of Mental Health (Sarason, 1977). World War II was truly a world war, and it was a long one. No one in this country was unaffected by the war. For millions of people family life was disrupted as one or more of a family's members (sons, fathers, close relatives) were gone for months or years, died, or came back a casualty or stranger. And many who remained at home also changed and were as strangers to the returning veterans. It was a mammoth upheaval that accelerated the pace of prewar, socially centrifugal forces of change. In films, novels, plays, and radio dramas there was a common message: As a result of the war, the world, and everyone in it, would never be the same. That was "good" because it meant that the opportunity to build a better world was at hand, but it also raised the question of whether people were appropriately prepared for the coming changes. Although the end of the war was greeted with ecstatic relief, it was also accompanied by anxiety about another economic depression, the readjustment of veterans to civilian life, and whether the government could move quickly enough to mount programs that would head off social unrest.

By saying that World War II ushered in the Age of Mental Health, I am trying to reflect several facts. One was the influential role of mental health professionals in the corridors of power and policy, roles undreamed of in the prewar period. If they gained such roles, it was in large part because there was in the larger society an inchoate consensus that the frequency of personal problems had escalated and would continue to do so. If the incidence of personal breakdowns among veterans during the war was disturbingly high, if the incidence would increase with war's end as veterans returned to civilian life, it followed that a large segment of the civilian population would be subjected to disabling stress. A health policy for veterans alone would not be adequate to deal with the nonveteran population. Viewed in this way, it was obvious that a crash program to train more mental health professionals would be needed. But, the mental health professionals said, there was not only a shortage of personnel but a shortage of scientific knowledge about the causes and treatment of personal disorders. What the government had to do, they said, was to support basic research. If the atomic scientists had contributed so much to the successful prosecution of the war, it was because they were able to exploit the findings of basic research. What the government had to recognize was that in the coming decades the frequency of disabling personal problems would emerge near or at the top of society's problems and unless more basic knowledge about human behavior was obtained, there was no telling what the consequences would be. These were the considerations that led to the annual increases in the budget of the National Institute of Mental Health (NIMH). The mental health professionals promised a lot, wanted a lot, and got a lot. I need not elaborate on the fact that psychiatry dominated in the formulation of NIMH policy and obtained the largest fraction of financial support. The social sciences were deemed important but in terms of expenditures, not all that important. In the case of NIMH training grants for clinical psychology, they were dispensed by criteria which required that clinical psychologists obtain their field training in medical–psychiatric settings.

The Age of Psychotherapy is another way to label the post-World War II years. From the standpoint of psychology as a field, it really began with the publication of Rogers's (1942) *Counseling and Psychotherapy*, a book that had quite an impact in and beyond psychology. This book was truly a pioneer effort, and I in no way intend to devalue it when I say that from my standpoint its consequences for clinical psychology and public policy were unfortunate. For one thing it defined (and made extraordinarily interesting) the problems of people in terms of an individual psychology: Problems were personal or narrowly interpersonal and for all practical purposes independent of the nature and structure of the social order. The mode of treatment was an individual one, which started a lively controversy about the comparative efficacy of different modes of individual treatment. Psychotherapy became the mental aspirin and people flocked to get the credentials to dispense it. The problem for public policy was how to train enough psychotherapists to deal with the people who needed them. But that problem ran headlong into another policy issue: Who owned psychotherapy? This issue is implied in the title of Rogers's book because if counseling and psychotherapy were basically the same, medicine and psychiatry could not claim, as they did, that these were only in their domain.

Anyone who lived through those days will testify to the vehemence and resources with which organized medicine and psychiatry fought to keep others from their turf. Organized psychiatry was faced with a problem in large measure of its own making. It had helped formulate and promote a public policy that recognized the need for clinical psychologists in the psychiatric setting, albeit in a subordinate role. But in terms of the overwhelming need for psychologists in these settings, on what basis could one deny clinical psychologists a therapeutic function? And even if one wanted to restrict psychologists to a diagnostic and research role, how could one deny them a function that would make those roles more cogent and effective? The battle was waged on legal, professional, and social grounds. It was also waged on financial and status grounds because about the only thing that was clear in the smoke of battle was that in the psychiatric setting there was a near perfect correlation between salary and status, on the one hand, and who did how much psychotherapy, on the other hand. But one other thing was clear: Psychiatric–medical settings were not created by and administered for nonmedical personnel.

One would be very wrong if one interpreted all that I have said as a diatribe against medicine and psychiatry. But one would be right in interpreting what I have said, ableit too briefly and oversimplified, as a way of describing characteristics of the culture of American medicine in our society. It is a culture that socializes its members to view themselves and others in isolating ways; it cannot countenance challenges to its conceptions of leadership; it is quintessentially clinically oriented in contrast to a preventive orientation; it operates on the principle that what is good for medicine is good for the society; and it is almost totally lacking in the sense of social history that makes one humble before the fact that as individuals and collectivities we are inevitably prisoners of time and place, that self-interest and public interest should not be assumed to be identical, that how self-interest is defined depends on where one is in the social order and that to transcend time and place, even in small part, requires that one put into words what the socialization process, because it was so effective, made it unnecessary to verbalize. I could, of course, say many positive things about American medicine, but to understand public policy in regards to illness—which means how, as a professional culture, it tries to influence the use and direction of society's resources —one has to look at American medicine in terms ot its traditions, institutional structures, rites of passage, and economic base and interests. It is trivializing the issue to discuss it in terms of the "good guys and the bad guys," a Manichean view derived from an individual psychology that leads to premature moralizing.

THE NARROW DIRECTION OF CLINICAL PSYCHOLOGY

Now let me turn to clinical psychology and why it took the directions it did. What factors led it, unfortunately from my standpoint, to become embroiled in the culture of American medicine and psychiatry? To do justice to this question would require writing a book. Here I briefly discuss only a few of the major facets of my answer. To begin, the clinical tradition had a very flimsy base in pre-war American psychology. At best psychology was aclinical in orientation; at worst, it was anticlinical. That is to say, psychology had no experience with what was involved in training clinical psychologists, with the creation of settings for clinical practice, and with the culture of existing settings devoted to clinical service. It was a Johnny-come-lately to the clinical scene. When, as a direct result of the experience of leading psychologists during the war, as well as of the stimulus provided by an emerging federal policy, psychology sought (and was sought) formally to enter the clinical scene, it self-consciously had and proclaimed two assets, one major and one minor. The major asset was its research traditions and sophistication. The minor asset was embedded in psychology's role in the testing movement. I call it a minor asset because the area of testing was never in the mainstream of American psychology, but was a tributary, and also because so much of what went on in testing was either nonclinical in goal or very superficially clinical. (It could be argued that, major or minor, psychology's contribution to the testing movement has had negative consequences for society.) These two assets were also highly regarded by psychiatry, which, in propagandizing (used here nonpejoratively) for a new public mental health policy, emphasized the need for research on diagnosis and treatment. Psychology may have come late to the scene, but it was cordially welcomed. It presented no challenge, conceptually and institutionally, to psychiatry. Psychology would be part of the team. There was no question about who would captain the team and where the game would be played.

I must digress here to mention another asset, far more subtle than the first two, that was fateful for the future. It was an asset (more in the nature of a mixed blessing) that was as overlooked as it was obvious, but it had the kind of obviousness the significance of which could only be appreciated if one looked at psychology in terms of its institutional placement and culture. I refer to the fact that psychology was an arts and science discipline, not a professional one, in the university. It had successfully fought for and obtained an independent status in the university, which is another way of saying that it was constituted of fiercely independent individuals encouraged to do and used to doing things their way. The socialization process in graduate education inculcated the values of autonomy and no-holds-barred pursuit of knowledge. The spirit of accommodation, let alone subordination, was not in the picture. Of course, this spirit was not in the picture in psychiatry and medicine either. Two subcultures were on a collision course, but like in so many partnerships and marriages, the characteristics that can produce collisions are rarely confronted despite their obviousness.

From the standpoint of psychology, the tie that was being forged between clinical psychology and the psychiatric setting was a socially responsible one. Psychology saw itself as meeting social needs in ways consistent with and enriching of its own traditions and knowledge. What was also attractive about this tie was that it would be financially underwritten by the federal government, meaning that students would be supported, faculties enlarged, and consultantships arranged. Were it not for federal policy and funds, would clinical psychology have forged the tie that it did? And if this question had been clearly raised, the truly important policy question for psychology would have to come to the fore: What was the universe of alternatives that psychology, in general, and clinical psychology, in particular, should consider in deciding how they could best contribute to what was defined as a staggering mental health problem? This was the question psychology had to ask in arriving at a policy. But the question was never seriously raised for several reasons. One is that psychology had no conceptual and research tradition in regard to policy formulation. Psychology had a long tradition of research on problem solving, but the significance of this tradition for the process of policy formulation was not seen. Another reason is that psychology, no less than psychiatry and medicine, was a babe-in-the-woods when it came to understanding the history and nature of government. This is but another way of saying that social psychology had never come to grips with the history, culture, and organization of American society. Social psychology was social in the sense that it was riveted on individuals and interactions among them: the attitudes individuals brought with them and the ways attitudes changed as a consequence of the interactions. It was social in the sense of having an interpersonal or a small-group focus. It was not social in the sense of placing these interactions in the context of a highly differentiated society with a distinctive culture and ideology that were reflected in and reinforced by governmental, political, educational, religious, and financial (profit-making) systems of institutions. This is the point that John Dewey made in his presidential address to the American Psychological Association in 1899 (see Hilgard, 1978). It is a point also made by Brown (1936) in his book *Psychology and the Social Order*, a heroically systematic effort to conceptually integrate Marx, Freud, and Lewin and a massive indictment of academic social psychology as well. Brown's book was the only social psychology text of the time to deal with the significance of the Great Depression. And more than passing mention must be made of Dollard's (1935) *Criteria for the Life History*, a title that unfortunately does not reflect what Dollard was about, which was to examine case descriptions of major theorists to see how seriously they took the concepts of culture and social order in relation to socialization and development. Dollard (1935) wrote,

> A life historian, sophisticated in the above sense, can see his life history subject as a link in a chain of social transmission; there were links before him from which he acquired his present culture; other links will follow him to which he will pass on the current of tradition. The life history attempts to describe a unit in that process; it is a study of one of the strands of a complicated collective life which has historical continuity. The fact that an individual believes his culture to be "his" in some powerful personal sense, as though he had thought out for himself how to do the things which he actually does by traditional prescription, will not impress the observer who has the cultural view. He will regard this conviction as unimportant and will stress the point of uniformity of the subject's behavior with that of persons who have lived before him and who now live in the same group. In such a "march" of a culture through time the individual is seen as less than a phantom; in point of fact, the individual only appears in times of crisis when the mores are not adequate to meet some real life situation which the group faces.

> *We are stressing at this point the fact that the scientific student of a human life must adequately acknowledge the enormous background mass of the culture; and not as a mere mass either, but rather as a configurated whole. Before any individual appears his society has had a specific social life organized and systematized, and the existence of this life will exercise a tyrannical compulsion on him. Seen from this point of view the problem of the life history is a statement of how the new organism becomes the victim or the resultant of this form structure of the culture.* Each life history that is gathered will be a record of how a new person is added to the group. It will be a case of seeing "the group plus a person." To state the point in an extreme manner we can think of the organic man as the mere toy of culture, providing it with a standardized base, investing its forms with affect but creating very little that is new alone or at any one time.
>
> If our life historian is not equipped with the above criterion he will certainly fall into error by referring to accident, whims of individuals, or organic propulsion, much that is properly seen only as a part of the society into which the individual comes. These errors seem so chronic and immortal in social science thinking that it is hard to overdo the necessity of a very schematic statement of the cultural view. *Many individuals who are quite able to state the point, after one fashion or another, are persistently unable to work it through into their manner of dealing with problems. One of the marks of an effective grasping of this point is the stated or implied "in our culture" whenever one makes any point in connection with individual behavior; it is a good thing to get into the habit, for example, of saying "men are more able than women to exhibit aggressive behavior in our culture." One might venture that to the social psychologist the three most indispensable letters in the alphabet are I.O.C. (in our culture).* (pp. 15–17, italics added)

Although Dollard found the clinical case descriptions inadequate by the criteria he employed, it would be a mistake to see his book only as a contribution to the clinical area. A close reading would convince the reader that Dollard—a sociologist, psychoanalyst, anthropologist, and psychologist—was indicting an asocial and acultural psychology.

It is hard to overestimate the consequences for clinical psychology of the lack of a foundation in a social psychology oriented, at least in part, to the nature of American society. There was nothing in American psychology that would have put on clinical psychology's agenda the role of women, the social class bias of the mental health movement, a similar bias in connection with all health services, the history of racial, religious, and ethnic discrimination, and perhaps most bothersome of all, the lack of a self-consciousness among psychologists that they were largely male, white, economically secure, and urbanized. One would be hard put to find evidence that in those days psychology knew that millions of people still lived in rural areas; one would be pardoned if one concluded from this that rural people were psychologically more hardy than their urban counterparts.

I said earlier that in serving as a matchmaker between clinical psychology and the psychiatric–medical setting, psychology was trying to meet the needs of society in ways that would be mutually beneficial. If this is true, how then can one explain that so many departments favored the tie with the VA even though their students would not see children or women? From the standpoint of theory and practice, as well as of the generality of research findings, how could psychology benefit from such parochialism? There are two parts to the answer: Psychology did not explore the universe of alternatives available to it, and few things rival money on the table in its capacity to short-circuit imagination. A fettered imagination impoverishes awareness of the universe of alternatives. Psychology was so focused on the money behind the proposed programs—in part because it served both narrow and socially desirable goals—that it totally failed to ask *the* question, If there was no money powering the invitation for clinical psychology to become part of the medical–psychiatric team, would psychology have moved in that direction? I submit that the failure to ask and examine this question was the hallmark of psychology's naiveté about itself and the social world in which it was embedded. The fact is that clinical psychology could have taken directions different from those it did. I am not saying that these directions were equally desirable and practical but, rather, that they were options that could have been considered. I could argue that from the standpoint of tradition and expertise, it would have made little difference which direction (or combination of directions) psychology took; it would in any event learn as it went along. It could, of course, have done nothing, as was the case in Canada, where after World War II psychiatry helped form a public policy that had no need of clinical psychology.

I would not be stressing the concept of the universe of alternatives if I did not believe that tying clinical psychology to the psychiatric setting was a major mistake from which clinical psychology continues to suffer. Clinical psychology became part of a medically dominated mental health movement that was narrow in terms of theory and settings, blind to the nature of the social order, and as imperialistic as it was vigorous. At least three generations of clinical psychology students became veterans of the war with psychiatry. Many had service-connected disabilities, but rather than ask for benefits, they preferred to leave and stay away from the battleground. There were more local battles and more Versailles-like peace conferences than some of us care to remember. And, of course, the superpowers—the American

Psychological Association and the American Psychiatric Association —took over and the local skirmishes were eclipsed in importance by superpower collisions in the courts, the legislatures, and the executive branches of state and federal government. Wars rarely, if ever, have the consequences the combatants envision. Clinical psychology did not fight the war to become like psychiatry (as it is now tending to be), that is, exclusive, money oriented, a lobbying force, supersensitive and superpious about upholding standards and monitoring credentials, and tolerant but not respectful of the research endeavor. It is a classic case, if I may momentarily resort to an individual psychology, of identification with the aggressor, a process as revealing as it is unconscious. I do not say this sneeringly but, rather, despairingly. By tying clinical psychology to the psychiatric setting, both sides put themselves on a collision course with each other. Clinical psychology—the young David to the big Goliath—needed more than a slingshot. It had to show that it was more protective of the public welfare, more concerned with quality, more concerned with credentialing and standards. The war was fought on psychiatry's grounds around issues primarily determined by the medical and psychiatric traditions.

THE SIGNIFICANCE OF THE BOULDER CONFERENCE

And now I must turn to the 1950 Boulder Conference (see Raimy, 1959) that was so fateful in determining the directions clinical psychology would take. Boulder was fateful not because it moved clinical psychology in new directions, but because it legitimated an orientation that had already been established during and immediately after the war. Boulder was sponsored by the Veterans Administration and the National Institute of Mental Health, a not unimportant fact because it indicates what outcomes were expected, if not in detail then in broad outline. As conferences go, and they rarely really *go,* Boulder was exceptional in terms of length, seriousness, level of intellectual discussion, and pursuit of goals. There was an unusual self-consciousness about the fact that a new field was being shaped which would impact on society and psychology as a field. The outcome was not surprising in terms of tying clinical psychology to medical–psychiatric settings, but this was not because the conference discussion did not permit challenges to its main thrust. It was as open a conference as has ever been held. Every criticism and reservation I voiced earlier about tying clinical psychology to the psychiatric setting was explicitly brought up at the conference.

I was at the conference as a young, upstart, nontenured associate professor who was inevitably in awe of the well-known, influential psychologists who were there. During graduate school at Clark University, I had had an externship at Worcester State Hospital, which was one of the few places (in my opinion, the only place) where there was real intellectual substance to what was then clinical psychology. But I also learned at Worcester State Hospital what it meant to be a second-class citizen in a psychiatric setting. If I had any doubts on this score, they evaporated after I took my first job at a new educationally oriented institution that had no psychiatrists and the superintendent of which, an educator, had been appointed over the most strenuous objections of the medical community. So coming from these experiences to Yale, and representing Yale at Boulder, I had strong convictions about tying clinical psychology to the medical-psychiatric setting. We were, I believed, not only asking for trouble but walking into a fight with chin out, hands down, and blurred vision. Why must the internship be in a psychiatric setting? Would psychology be capitalizing on its research traditions if clinical students were unsophisticated in psychotherapy? How could one justify the clinical emphasis at the expense of a preventive orientation? Would not psychology be more responsive to societal needs if it made a commitment to the public schools? Why should clinical psychology be tied to a setting that would not expose its members to such areas as mental retardation, criminality, physical handicap, and vocational planning and adjustment? Why was the curriculum that was being outlined weighed in favor of such elective courses as neurophysiology, pharmacology, and neuroanatomy? These issues were raised and joined, and the outcome was predictable. Only a handful of people at Boulder took the position I did. I do not think I ever expressed it at Boulder, but I know the following thought crossed my mind: If the funding for the development of clinical psychology was coming from other sources with no strings attached, would clinical psychology move in the direction it was going? In some vague way I knew that the conference was not confronting the age-old maxim that the hand that feeds you is the hand that can starve you, that money as an incentive is almost always powerful and frequently and unwittingly corrupting. And by corrupting I mean that dependence, in whole or in part, on a funding source facilitates rationalizations that constrict one's thinking about alternatives more congruent with one's initial values, expectations, and capabilities. The problem is made more difficult when one is part of a professional field, the internal policies of which reinforce the tie with the external funding source.

By virtue of the nature and details of the origins of modern clinical psychology, it is not surprising that one of the characteristics of its development has been concern with achieving independence from and a kind of parity with psychiatry. This concern catapulted the field into the arenas of politics, legislation, lobbying, and public policy. It was a move to gain and preserve independence, not to change the conceptual substance of mental health policy. It was a move to be considered as good as and as financially deserving as "them." It was not a move that challenged the underlying conceptions of public policy, for example, its focus on the individual organism deriving from an asocial psychology. Nor was it a move that stemmed from an attempt to identify past conceptual mistakes but, rather, one that recognized past organizational mistakes. Self-scrutiny has never been a notable characteristic of professional organizations. I should amend this statement, however, by saying that professional organizations do scrutinize their political–organizational mistakes, but only when their status is threatened. The recognition that a field may have based itself on faulty conceptions of the nature of its subject matter always reflects sea-swell changes in the society, impacting on the field along a time dimension quite different from our usual experience of time.

Now to an instructive anecdote that illustrates how we can be unfortunate prisoners of time and place unless our education builds into us schemata that aid us in taking distance from our time and place. One not only has always to say "in our culture" (Dollard, 1935) but to add "at this time and place." This anecdote relates to a future condition that already existed in the present but to which no one was paying heed. If the cast of characters had had the conceptual tools to help them divorce themselves from the compelling quality of their concrete present, clinical psychology might not have made the kinds of commitments it did. The anecdote is about a meeting that took place either shortly before or shortly after the Boulder Conference. I do not remember the point of the occasion or the names of most of the dozen or so people who were there. I do know that there were representatives of university clinical training programs and staff from the regional and central VA offices. At one point a VA staff person said, "Do you realize that the young veterans we are talking about will someday be old veterans, and we have a lot of those now from World War I, and we will not have the appropriate knowledge or facilities?" Nobody, including myself, responded to his comments and the meeting went on, probably to rehash the problems of training clinical psychologists. But it is as if his words were seared on my brain. I knew that what he said was important, but it took years for me to appreciate the wisdom of his words. I would like to believe that he understood, like no one else at the meeting, the difference between preventive and clinical thinking. His totally uninfluential comments were, or course, confirmed in subsequent years: The VA is now responsible for more geriatric cases than any other societal agency—responsible but unprepared.

The point of the anecdote, thus, is that after World War II a health policy was being forged that was narrow in scope, not grounded in an attempt to conceptualize the nature of society and its social order, amazingly ahistorical, and resting on the belief that the future would be a carbon copy of the present. It was a policy forged by professionals who had no way of asking, How are the ways we are defining problems and modes of attack a function of where *we* are in the social order? How should awareness of our place in the social order serve as a warning that we are subject to certain biases and distortions in regard to our society and its needs? How does our place in its social order—the result of a host of selective factors which interact with a distinctive, prolonged education that emphasizes how different we are from the rest of society—prevent us from recognizing that, like it or not, we are part of the problem because we are in the stream of social history? One cannot ask these kinds of questions without being realistically humble. Humbleness is not a word that easily comes to mind when one reviews the mental health movement after World War II. Personal, intellectual, and professional arrogance comes more quickly to mind. The roots that clinical psychology had in American psychology were shallow, but they at least contained the fertilizing ingredient of skepticism. But that ingredient came only from an individual psychology, and it was (and still is) inadequately sustaining when psychology, in general, and clinical psychology, in particular, entered the arena of social reality and public policy. In those arenas an individual psychology is a mammoth distraction.

The therapeutic endeavor needs no justification, but when that endeavor becomes nearly all-encompassing in focus and policy, one must suspect not only the crippling role of parochial thinking but also the failure to examine and confront the nature of the society itself. A clinical psychology not rooted in a realistic social psychology —that is, a social psychology which sees itself as a cultural and social-historical product and agent, which sees itself by virtue of time, place, and social and institutional status as both a cultural cause and a cultural effect—is a misdirected clinical psychology. This point has been recognized by others of my generation who grew up in clinical psychology and none has said it better than Cowen (1980) in his recent stimulating article on primary prevention. Cowen is too realistic to be other than humble about our knowledge of how to approach primary prevention. As a clinician he knows how a part of us, as individuals, needs and treasures our symptoms, and as a community psychologist he knows how refractory our communities have been and will be to the efforts at primary prevention. He also knows that going the route of primary prevention will illuminate not only important features of the social order but also how those features will be obstacles to mounting effective programs in primary prevention. And he also knows that psychology will vigorously resist changing its dependence on an individual psychology.

I sense a breeze of change in psychology's air. The October 1979 issue of the *American Psychologist*, a special issue, was devoted to "Psychology and Children: Current Research and Practice." One of the articles is as incisive as it is brief. It was written by an eminent child developmentalist, William Kessen. Kessen's (1979) comments about what is wrong in child psychology are similar to what Cowen and I have said. American psychology, invented in and by American society, went on to invent its subject matter: the self-contained individual. The necessity for reinvention is at hand. Necessity may be the mother of invention, but let us never forget that inventions are rarely unmixed blessings.

Nothing in what I have said, and nothing in what Cowen and Kessen have said, denies that individual psychologies have contributed to our knowledge of human behavior and development. And, it should go without saying, nothing in what I have said in this article should in any way be interpreted as subordinating one approach (e.g., biological) to another. It is precisely the subordination of one approach to another that I have argued against. Anyone who is familiar with the past and current status of departments of public health in medical schools—or the sad fate of departments of community medicine—will be familiar with the adverse institutional and social consequences of subordinating one approach to another in the health area. Human illness and misery have diverse sources within and without the individual. If only because of this glimpse of the obvious, we must radically reexamine how we conceptualize the individual organism. This reexamination is crucial if we are to deepen our understanding and direct more effectively our capacities to prevent and repair.

The shortcomings of extant psychologies would not have been exposed in the way they have if psychology had remained a narrow, university-based, and encapsulated discipline. But the world—our entire, globe-straddling social world—changed and psychology was drawn into it as never before. To understand individuals for the purpose of influencing or helping them is one thing. To understand and influence social orders for the purpose of influencing parts of them is another thing, even if what one seeks to influence is a particular service to individuals. Ultimately, both types of understanding and the actions derived from them have to be conceptually interrelated because in the real world they are interrelated. The shortcomings of clinical psychology were inherent in those of American psychology. By emphasizing the short-comings of clinical psychology, I have run the risk of blaming the victim. My aim has not been to blame victim or aggressor because to do so would be to trivialize the matter by resort to what Mills (1959) called unwarranted and misleading "psychologisms" deriving from an individual psychology. There is a creeping sense of malaise in psychology about psychology. But that malaise is not peculiar to psychology. It is suffusing the atmosphere in all the social sciences. Indeed, in some of the social sciences, like economics, there are those who not only believe that the emperor is naked but also that he has a terminal disease. But this kind of medical metaphor, however apt it may seem, is but another example of how our thinking is imprisoned in an individual psychology.

REFERENCES

Brown, J. F. *Psychology and the social order*. New York: McGraw-Hill, 1936.

Cowen, E. L. The wooing of primary prevention. *American Journal of Community Psychology*, 1980, *8*, 258–284.

Dollard J. *Criteria for the life history*. New Haven, Conn.: Yale University Press, 1935.

Hilgard, E. (Ed.). *American psychology in historical perspective*. Washington, D.C.: American Psychological Association, 1978.

Kessen, W. The American child and other cultural inventions. *American Psychologist*, 1979, *34*, 815–820.

Mills, C. W. *The sociological imagination*. New York: Oxford University Press, 1959.

Raimy, V. C. (Ed.). *Training in clinical psychology*. Englewood Cliffs, N.J.: Prentice-Hall, 1950.

Rogers, C. R. *Counseling and psychotherapy*. Boston: Houghton Mifflin, 1942.

Sarason, S. B. *Work, aging, and social change. Professionals and the one life–one career imperative*. New York: Free Press, 1977.

Sarason, S. B. *Psychology misdirected*. New York: Free Press, 1981.

16
Autobiography

The most pervasive influences in my personal life were my family, the Great Depression, and polio, the last leaving me with limited use of my right arm. The fact that I was Jewish played a special role, which is described earlier in this book. In a brief biographical sketch such as this, it is obviously impossible, indeed inappropriate, to try to elaborate on the strength and direction of these influences. Suffice it to say that I have long felt marginal in my profession and in our society; that is, I have felt more an outsider than an insider—a stance conducive to dissent, self-probing, and the desire-ambition to change the world.

My undergraduate education (1935-39) was at Dana College, which became the University of Newark and much later became the Newark campus of Rutgers University. Dana was a liberating, exciting place, with a faculty unrivaled for its capacity to open new vistas for its students, all of whom were commuters. I had two psychology instructors: Fred Gaudet and Bob Watson. They taught everything from the Purkinje phenomenon to the ceremonial rites of the Kwakuitl Indians of the Pacific Northwest. Between these extremes were the more traditional topics. Bob Watson was getting his doctorate from Columbia (where Fred also had received his degree) and I was mightily impressed with his knowledge, although I do not recall that he then had the interest in history that later was the basis for his major contribution to the field.

I wanted to go to law school. What else could a nice, Jewish boy do if he could not go to medical school? Besides, Fred had done his dissertation on individual differences in the sentencing tendency of judges, and I was assisting him (thanks to the National Youth Administration) in some further legal research. When I became a senior and it was obvious that I could not afford to go to law school—and psychology had come to have more allure than law—I applied to graduate school with the hope that I would be awarded a fellowship. I think I applied to thirteen schools (including Yale, Harvard School of Education, Wisconsin), and twelve turned me down. My formal credentials were not outstanding: a B+ or A– average, the 75th percentile on the Henmon-Nelson intelligence test, and my college, which had just received accreditation. I was admitted to Clark University, which paid for tuition ($300) and a stipend of $200. Clark had undergone drastic changes—Walter Hunter going to Brown and other luminaries going elsewhere. In contrast to its past, the department was in a bad way. They must have had trouble attracting graduate students—the only explanation for why they took me. Clark was wonderful to me and for me. Saul Rosenzweig from the Worcester State Hospital, who taught abnormal psychology, mightily influenced me in that course and in connection with my thesis, for which he was my major advisor. Don Super was another influence, as was R. B. Cattell, who represented a very distinctive way of looking at psychological issues. I learned much about the eye and the ear from Robert Brown, enough to know that I was not cut out to be a sensory psychologist. During my second year, Charlotte and Karl Bühler were visiting professors who were intellectually and interpersonally very instructive. Recent generations of psychologists may be unfamiliar with the Bühlers, but each of them, especially Karl, made lasting contributions to their fields.

Clark was intimidating in one respect: *the* seminar room (in those days you needed only one seminar room) had pictures of everyone who had taught there or who had received doctorates there. It may be comforting to know that you are standing on the shoulders of giants, but it is intimidating to have them staring at you. Are there psychologists today who do not know the role of Clark University in American psychology?

I am not being maudlin or indulging in oily sentiment when I note that it was at Clark that I met Esther Kroop, who later became my wife. No one has been more important to me in my adult life. When I say important, I mean it both personally and intellectually. The major changes in direction in my professional career, in one or another way, were partly caused by her influence. In our society, life (in or out of academia) is not easy, and Esther's selflessness and unconditional support, for which she has paid a price in her professional endeavors, were incalculably important to me—a debt that gets larger with the years.

I was the first student at Clark to be allowed to do an externship at Worcester State Hospital, thanks to Saul Rosenzweig and David

Shakow. The department of psychology at the Worcester State Hospital stands in the same relationship to modern clinical psychology as Clark stands in relationship to American psychology. I write these words a week after David's death, and I am sorry that this is the first occasion I have had to acknowledge in print what the field owes him. David Shakow was a central node in a network of people from the various social sciences who gave substance and direction to the interrelationships among clinical psychology, psychoanalysis, and social science. When I decided I needed to be psychoanalyzed, it was David who sent me to Bela Mittelman, saying "He will not be hard on you." That says as much about David as it does about Bela Mittelman.

From Clark I went as chief psychologist to the Southbury Training School in Connecticut. Earlier in this book I have discussed the significance of those years at Southbury and my move to Yale.

I have been unusually fortunate in having friends and collaborators who, in similar and different ways, stimulated and advanced my thinking and knowledge. Thomas Gladwin opened up the field of cultural anthropology to me in ways that have been lastingly useful. More than that, his own changes in orientation toward the social sciences and our society kept me from forgetting (at least some of the time) that you pay a heavy intellectual price for being part of the establishment. Henry Schaefer-Simmern a political refugee from Hitler's Germany, an art theorist and art historian—not only nurtured me in art and the artistic process but also taught me the psychological and social meanings of the concept of the Gestalt. Despite the marked disparity in our ages, we were intellectual colleagues for almost four decades, until his recent death. He was a model of courage, independence, and knowledge that emboldened me to do what I felt I had to do. Burton Blatt—who has no peer when it comes to guts, sensitivity, and decency—broadened my knowledge of education and mental retardation and in countless ways helped me stay in touch with the dilemmas of the real world. His career is a good example of how one can try to change the world without trampling on the needs and feelings of others. John Doris (another fiercely independent soul), with whom I have collaborated the most, deeply influenced my knowledge of and excitement with intellectual and social history. How eagerly I would open up the package containing his latest chapters on social history and mental retardation to read the fascinating nuggets he had uncovered somewhere in the Cornell library. Wendell Garner—a splendid example of how one must distinguish between appearance and reality in human relationships—is the wisest person I have ever known. No one in American psychology understands better the theory-practice interrelationships. His scientific credentials are both impeccable and unrivaled, matched only by his knowledge of how the social world is organized and how it works.

I am a voracious, semi-indiscriminate reader, the major consequence of which has been getting acquainted with writers in diverse fields who helped me overcome the parochialism inevitable in one's own training. Roger Barker, John Dollard (sociologist, anthropologist, psychoanalyst, psychologist), Robert Nisbet, Edward Sapir, Isaiah Berlin, John Dewey, Ignazio Silone, Edmund Wilson, Lewis Mumford, Leon Trotsky, J. F. Brown—this is a very small sample of the writers who expanded my horizons. In the strict sense of the meanings of the terms, I am neither scholar nor researcher. Two decades ago I realized that I was temperamentally unable to take *a* problem and stick with it over a period of time. I used to feel guilty about that, as if I had to justify my existence by being truly expert, substantively and methodologically, about an area of problem. I no longer feel guilty, but I continue to be sad because I know that, at the end of my days, I will not have perused every book in the Yale library. The major problems of living are not soluble in the scientific sense of solution!

Publications: A Comprehensive Bibliography

1943

1. The use of the thematic apperception test with mentally deficient children: I. *American Journal of Mental Deficiency* 47:4.
2. The use of the thematic apperception test with mentally deficient children: II. *American Journal of Mental Deficiency* 48: 169-173.

1944

1. Dreams and thematic apperception test stories. *Journal of Abnormal and Social Psychology* 39:4.
2. Projective techniques in mental deficiency. *Journal of Personality*, pp. 237-245.
3. With Schaefer-Simmern, H. Therapeutic implications of artistic activity. A case study. *American Journal of Mental Deficiency* 49: 185-196.

1945

With Sarason, E. K. A problem in diagnosing feeblemindedness. *Journal of Abnormal and Social Psychology* 40: 323-329.

1947

1. With Boehm, A. E. Does Wechsler's formula distinguish intellectual deterioration from mental deficiency? *Journal of Abnormal and Social Psychology* 42(3).
2. With Potter, E. N. Color in the Rorschach and Kohs block designs. *Journal of Consulting Psychology* 11(4): 202-206.
3. With Sarason, E. K. The discriminatory value of a test pattern in the high grade familial defective. *Journal of Clinical Psychology* 3: 141-147.

1948

The TAT and subjective interpretation. *Journal of Consulting Psychology* 12 (5): 285-299.

1949

1. *Psychological problems in mental deficiency* (1st ed). New York: Harper and Brothers.
2. With Wittenborn, J. R. Exceptions to certain Rorschach criteria of pathology. *Journal of Consulting Psychology* 13(1): 21-27.

1950

The test-situation and the problem of prediction. *Journal of Clinical Psychology* 6(4): 378–392.

1951

1. Mental subnormality and the behavioral sciences. *Journal of Exceptional Children*, pp. 243–247.
2. The psychologist's behavior as an area of research. *Journal of Consulting Psychology* 15(4): 278–280.

1952

1. Aspects of a community program for the retarded child. *The Training School Bulletin* (Vineland, N. J.), pp. 201–207.
2. Individual psychotherapy with mentally defective individuals. *American Journal of Mental Deficiency* 56(4): 803–805.
3. With Mandler, G. A study of anxiety and learning. *Journal of Abnormal and Social Psychology* 47(2): 166–173.
4. With Mandler, G. Some correlates of test anxiety. *Journal of Abnormal and Social Psychology* 47(4): 810–817.
5. With Mandler, G., & Craighill, P. G. The effect of differential instructions on anxiety and learning. *Journal of Abnormal and Social Psychology* 47(2): 561–565.

1953

1. The mentally defective child. In *Psychology of exceptional children and youth*, ed. W. Cruikshank. New York: Prentice-Hall.
2. With Gladwin, T. *Truk: Man in paradise*. New York: Viking Fund Publications in Anthropology.
3. With Gordon, E. M. The test anxiety questionnaire: Scoring norms. *Journal of Abnormal and Social Psychology* 48(3): 447–448.
4. With Mandler, G. The effect of prior experience and subjective failure on the evocation of test anxiety. *Journal of Personality* 21(3): 336–341.

1954

1. *The clinical interaction.* New York: Harper and Brothers.
2. With Cox, F. N. Test anxiety and Rorschach performance. *Journal of Abnormal and Social Psychology* 49: 371–377.

1955

1. With Doris, J. Test anxiety and blame assignment in a failure situation. *Journal of Abnormal and Social Psychology* 50(3): 335–358.
2. With Gordon, E. The relationship between test anxiety and other anxieties. *Journal of Personality* 23: 317–323.

1958

1. With Davidson, K. S., Lighthall, F. F., & Waite, R. R. A test anxiety scale for children. *Child Development* 29(March): 105–113.
2. With Davidson, K. S., Lighthall, F. F., & Waite, R. R. Classroom observations of high and low anxious children. *Child Development* 29(June): 287–295.
3. With Davidson, K. S., Lighthall, F. F., Waite, R. R., & Sarnoff, I. Differences between mothers' and fathers' ratings of low anxious and high anxious children. *Child Development* 29(March): 155–160.
4. With Davidson, K. S., & Waite, R. R. Rorschach behavior and performance of high and low anxious children. *Child Development* 29(June): 277–285.
5. With Fox, C., Davidson, K. S., Lighthall, F. F., & Waite, R. R. Human figure drawings of high and low anxious children. *Child Development* 29(June): 297–301.
6. With Gladwin, T. Psychological and cultural problems in mental subnormality. *Genetic Psychology Monographs* 57:3–290.
7. With Nasland, R. L., & Gladwin, T. *Mental subnormality.* New York: Basic Books.
8. With Sarnoff, I., Lighthall, F. F., Waite, R. R., & Davidson, K. S. A cross-cultural study of anxiety among American and English school children. *Journal of Educational Psychology* 49(3): 129–136.
9. With Waite, R. R., Lighthall, F. F., & Davidson, K. S. A study of anxiety and learning in children. *Journal of Abnormal and Social Psychology* 57(3): 267–270.

1959

1. With Lighthall, F. F., & Ruebush, B. K. Change in mental ability as a function of test anxiety and type of mental test. *Journal of Consulting Psychology* 23(1): 34–38.
2. With Sarnoff, I., Lighthall, F. F., & Davidson, K. S. Test anxiety and the "eleven-plus" examinations. *British Journal of Educational Psychology* 29(Pt. I): 9–16.

1960

1. With Davidson, K. S., Waite, R. R., Lighthall, F. F., & Ruebush, B. K. *Anxiety in elementary school children: A report of research.* New York: Wiley.
2. With Lighthall, F. F., Davidson, K. S., Waite, R. R., & Sarnoff, I. The effects of serial position and time interval on two anxiety questionnaires. *Journal of Genetic Psychology* 63: 113–131.

1961

1. The contents of human problem solving. In *Nebraska symposium on motivation*, pp. 147–178. Lincoln: University of Nebraska Press.

2. With Barnard, J. W., & Zimbardo, P. G. Anxiety and verbal behavior in children. *Child Development* 32: 379–392.
3. With Davidson, K. S. Test anxiety and classroom observations. *Child Development* 32: 199–210.

1962

With Davidson, K. S., & Blatt, B. *The preparation of teachers: An unstudied problem in education.* New York: Wiley.

1964

1. Some aspects of the brain-behavior problem. Paper presented at the Second National Northwest Summer Conference: The Special Child in Century 21. *Journal of Education* 147: 53–61.
2. With Hill, K. T., & Zimbardo, P. G. A longitudinal study of the relation of test anxiety to performance on intelligence and achievement tests. *Child Development Monographs* 29(7): 4–51.

1966

1. The nature and assessment of anxiety in children. In *Anxiety and behavior,* ed. C. D. Spielberger. New York: Academic Press.
2. The school culture and process of change. Brechbill Lecture presented at the University of Maryland, January.
3. With Hill, K. T. The relation of test anxiety and defensiveness to test and school performance over the elementary-school years: A further longitudinal study. *Child Development Monographs* 31(2): 1–75.
4. With Levine, M., Goldenberg, I. I., Cherlin, D., & Bennett, E. *Psychology in community settings: Clinical, educational, vocational, social aspects.* New York: Wiley.

1967

Towards a psychology of change and innovation. *American Psychologist* 22: 227–233.

1969

1. The creation of settings. In *The Yale Psycho-Educational Clinic: Papers and research studies,* ed. F. Kaplan and S. B. Sarason. Boston: Massachusetts State Department of Mental Health Monograph Series.
2. With Doris, J. *Psychological problems in mental deficiency,* 4th ed. New York: Harper & Row.

1971

The culture of the school and the problem of change. Boston: Allyn & Bacon.

1972

1. *The creation of settings and the future societies.* San Francisco: Jossey-Bass.
2. With Grossman, F. K., & Zitnay, G. *The creation of a community setting.* Syracuse: Syracuse University Press.

1973

1. Jewishness, blackishness, and the nature-nurture controversy. *American Psychologist* 28(November): 962–971.
2. Social action as a vehicle for learning. In *The helping professions in the world of action*, ed. I. I. Goldenberg. Lexington, Mass.: Lexington Books, D. C. Heath.

1974

The psychological sense of community: Prospects for a community psychology. San Francisco: Jossey-Bass.

1975

1. Psychology *To the Finland Station* in *The Heavenly City of the Eighteenth Century Philosophers. American Psychologist* 30(November): 1072–1080.
2. With Sarason, E. K., & Cowden, P. Aging and the nature of work. *American Psychologist* 30(May): 584–592.
3. With Study Team of the Institute for Responsive Education. The community at the bargaining table: A report on the community's role in collective bargaining in the schools. Boston: Institute for Responsive Education, January.

1976

1. Community psychology and the anarchist insight. *American Journal of Community Psychology* 4(3): 243–261.
2. Community psychology, networks, and Mr. Everyman. *American Psychologist* 31(May): 317–328.
3. Educational policy and federal intervention in the "days of opportunity." *Journal of Education* 158(4): 3–24.
4. The unfortunate fate of Alfred Binet and school psychology. *Teachers College Record* (Columbia University) 77 (May): 579–592.

1977

1. *Work, aging, and social change: Professionals and the one life–one career imperative.* New York: Free Press.
2. A "cultural" limitation of system approaches to educational reform. *American Journal of Community Psychology* 5(3): 277–287.
3. With Carroll, C., Maton, K., Cohen, S., & Lorentz, E. *Human services and resource networks.* San Francisco: Jossey-Bass.

1978

1. The nature of problem solving in social action. *American Psychologist* 33(April): 370–380.
2. An unsuccessful war on poverty? *American Psychologist* 33(September): 831–839.

1979

1. With Doris, J. *Educational handicap, public policy, and social history: A broadened perspective on mental retardation.* New York: Free press.
2. With Lorentz, E. *The challenge of the resource exchange network.* San Francisco: Jossey-Bass.

1980

1. Individual psychology: An obstacle to comprehending adulthood. In *Competence and coping during adulthood,* ed. L. A. Bond and J. C. Rosen. Hanover, N.H.: University Press of New England.
2. Review of Jensen, Bias in mental testing. *Society*, No. 1, pp. 86–88.

1981

1. Psychology misdirected: The psychologist in the social order. New York: Free Press.
2. An asocial psychology and a misdirected clinical psychology. *American Psychologist* 36(8): 827–836.

Author Index

Subject Index

Abnormal psychology, 254

Abstract: symbols, 73; truth, 141

Academic psychiatry, 239

Academic psychology, 196

Achievement tests, 16, 63–64, 68

Administration and administrators: functions of, 27, 144, 147, 155; school, 141, 182, 218; youth, 253

Adults and adulthood, 30, 52, 187, 218, 223, 228, 230

Age and aging: discrimination against, 81; and the elderly, 80–83, 89, 136; factor of, 23–24, 30, 216; groups, 31; and mental health, 6, 14, 224; process of, 95–96, 141, 218; programs, 83, 89; sense of, 77, 80–81, 84, 87; and youth, 187

Age of Mental Health (Sarason), 239–240

Agencies: community action, 165, 168; human service, 220; social service, 219

Aggressiveness, evidence of, 28–29, 245

Alcoholism, problem of, 18

Aloneness, sense of, 195

American Constitutional Convention, The, 45, 127

American Historical Association, 172

American Journal of Community Psychology, 135n, 177n

American Journal of Psychology, 122–124

American Psychiatric Association (APA), 162–163, 247

American Psychological Association (APA), 13n, 127, 161–162, 192, 233, 235, 236, 244, 246–247

American Psychologist, cited, 59n, 79n, 117n, 153n, 191n, 235n, 251n

American psychology, aspects of, 8, 12, 41, 43–44, 57, 115–116, 124, 127, 175, 189, 192, 211, 234–236, 250, 252, 255

American West, The: New Perspectives, New Dimensions (Steffen), 5

Anarchism and anarchists: factor of, 141, 143; ideology, 139–140; insight, 145–148

Anarchy and Order (Read), 140n

Anger, feelings of, 83

Animal instincts, 122

Anthropologists, 22, 156, 202, 229, 245, 256

Anthropology, 6; cultural, 255; data on, 47; departments of, 4

Anti-Defamation League of the B'nai Brith, 74

Anxiety: levels of, 16–20, 27–28, 55, 83–84, 112, 114, 153, 206, 219; research in, 22, 108. *See also* Test Anxiety Project

Apes, problem solving in, 192–193, 198

Applied psychology, 128

Armed Services programs, 11, 18. *See also* Veterans Administration (VA)

Arthur Performance Point Scale, 16–17

Asia, 60

Assessment centers, 24–27

Atomic scientists, 200, 202, 206, 229, 240

Atomism, clinical, 14

Attitudes: changes in, 60, 64, 67, 87; cultural, 74–75, 81; ethnic, 175; group, 59, 68; historically rooted, 64–65, 68–69, 73; hostile, 36; political, 66; racial, 70; realistic, 36–37; role of, 23–25, 28–29, 63, 91; toward self, 24, 28

Authenticity. *See* Truth and candor

Authority: centralized, 137; of nature, 125; school, 36

Ethics and moral questions, 104, 238
Ethnic attitudes and groups, 72–74, 175, 179, 245
Eugenics, field of, 70n
Europe, 60
Evolution, alleged theories of, 138
Existentialism, 46, 124
Experiences: children's educational, 39, 177–178, 182; learning, 25; personal, 81; religious, 124, 205
Experimental cognitive psychologists, 12
Exploratory studies, 86–88

Failure, aspects of, 18, 24, 29–30
Faith: capacity for, 126–127; decline in, 204–205; religious, 131
Family and familial relationships: behavior, 34; politics of, 170; problems, 18, 237; unit structure of, 37, 49, 84, 91, 218–219, 222, 238, 253
Fantasy, factor of, 28, 107
Fears. *See* Anxiety
Federal Administration on Aging, 83n
Federal programs, 51, 109, 136–138, 141–142, 147, 236, 243
Feeblemindedness, problem of, 14, 19
Finland Station, 118, 124, 131
Food stamps, 136
France, 129; revolution in, 126, 129
Freedom: intellectual, 101; personal, 214; traditions of, 65
Friendliness and familiarity, feelings of, 23, 28–29
Frustration, problem of, 18–19, 37, 85–86, 217–218
Funds, fees and funding, 141–142, 161, 181–182, 238, 243
Future of the United States, The (Orlans), 140

Genes, carriers of, 2, 57
Genetic processes, 57, 59, 68, 75, 131, 198
Genotypic characteristics, factor of, 5, 42, 145
Geography, influence of, 158
Gestalt, concept of, 14, 99n, 121, 160, 222, 255

Ghetto: children, 184; schools, 180
GI Bill, results of, 6. *See also* Veterans, readjustment policies
Goals, perception of, 33, 52, 105
God, feelings on, 125, 127
Graduate education, 4, 6, 87–88, 243; programs, 192, 216–217; school, 27, 66, 84–85, 97, 216, 219; students, 4, 26, 109
Grant programs and support of, 108–109, 141–142, 157, 225
Great Britain, 70n, 124
Great Depression, era of, 1, 96, 107, 135–139, 197, 202, 244, 253
Great Society program, 203n
Greek philosophy, 229
Group(s): age, 31; attitudes, 59, 68; black, 67; responses, 14; techniques, 46
Growing Up Old in The Sixties (Maynard), 82
Guilt feelings, absence of, 28

Handicapped persons, 1, 34, 37, 39
Harvard School of Education, 254
Head Start program, 51, 180, 183–184
Health service, 49, 133, 158, 238–240
Heavenly City of the Eighteenth Century Philosophers, The (Becker), 124–132
Hebrew: religion, 128; schools, 60
Henmon-Nelson intelligence test, 254
Hillel organization, 66
Historically rooted attitudes and groups, 64–65, 68–69, 73
History: of behaviorism, 194; case, 28; conception of, 12, 55, 57, 120; cultural, 58, 63, 72, 106; intellectual, 12; scientific, 115, 128n; social, 8, 58–59, 115, 151, 157, 175, 195, 197, 205–207, 233–237, 241–242, 255
Hospitals: general, 24; laboratory, 11, 16; mental, 24, 102, 220, 227; state, 19, 102, 146, 226; types of, 18, 51
Hostility, problem of, 36, 69
Human: behavior, 14, 47, 196, 240; history, 68, 119, 126–127; mind,